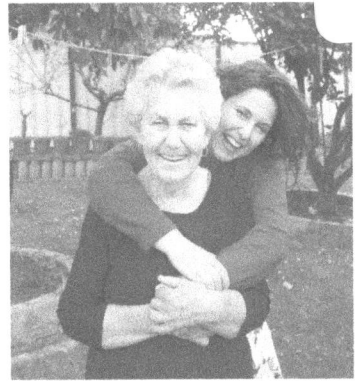

Spiri Tsintziras is an author, teacher, one-time social worker, mother, daughter, partner and writer of life stories.

Her mother, Chrisoula, has taught her about the life-giving benefits of laughter, tenacity, and how to eat with gusto. She continues to inspire many of Spiri's stories.

Twelve Golden Gifts is Spiri's third memoir, following *Afternoons in Ithaka* and *My Ikaria*.

Spiri lives in Melbourne with her family.

Also by Spiri Tsintziras

My Ikaria

Afternoons in Ithaka

Parlour Games for Modern Families (with Myfanwy Jones)

Twelve Golden Gifts

SPIRI TSINTZIRAS

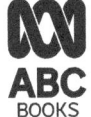
ABC
BOOKS

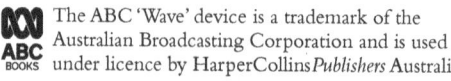 The ABC 'Wave' device is a trademark of the Australian Broadcasting Corporation and is used under licence by HarperCollins*Publishers* Australia

HarperCollins*Publishers*
Australia • Brazil • Canada • France • Germany • Holland • India
Italy • Japan • Mexico • New Zealand • Poland • Spain • Sweden
Switzerland • United Kingdom • United States of America

HarperCollins acknowledges the Traditional Custodians
of the lands upon which we live and work, and pays respect
to Elders past and present.

First published on Gadigal Country in Australia in 2025
by HarperCollins*Publishers* Australia Pty Limited
ABN 36 009 913 517
harpercollins.com.au

Copyright © Spiri Tsintziras 2025

The right of Spiri Tsintziras to be identified as the author of this work has been asserted by her in accordance with the *Copyright Act 1968*.

All rights reserved. Apart from any use as permitted under the *Copyright Act 1968*, no part may be reproduced, copied, scanned, stored in a retrieval system, recorded, or transmitted, in any form or by any means, without the prior written permission of the publisher. Without limiting the exclusive rights of any author, contributor, or the publisher of this publication, any unauthorised use of this publication to train generative artificial intelligence (AI) technologies is expressly prohibited. HarperCollins also exercises its rights under Article 4(3) of the Digital Single Market Directive 2019/790 and expressly reserves this publication from the text and data-mining exception

HarperCollins*Publishers*
Macken House, 39/40 Mayor Street Upper
Dublin 1, D01 C9W8, Ireland

A catalogue record for this book is available from the National Library of Australia

ISBN 978 0 7333 4374 2 (paperback)
ISBN 978 1 4607 1823 0 (ebook)

Cover design by Hazel Lam, HarperCollins Design Studio
Cover image by Adobe Stock
Author photograph by George Mifsud
Typeset in Adobe Garamond Pro by Kirby Jones

Printed and bound by CPI Group (UK) Ltd, Croydon, CR0 4YY

To my beautiful mother, Chrisoula
May your golden spirit continue to shine bright

Contents

Mamma — 1

Gift #1 Generosity — 3
Gift #2 Openness — 27
Gift #3 Humour — 51
Gift #4 Warmth — 67
Gift #5 Love — 85
Gift #6 Joy — 113
Gift #7 Humanity — 133
Gift #8 Persistence — 159
Gift #9 Understanding — 187
Gift #10 Kindness — 221
Gift #11 Compassion — 235
Gift #12 Spirit — 247
Epilogue — 275

Twelve carer lessons — 283
More information — 301
Permissions — 307
Acknowledgements — 309

Mamma

Mamma mou,
I sit down to write words that will do you justice. But my hands lie still, paralysed by the enormity of the task. The poor house of language is too small for your remarkable spirit.

I think of your name, *Mamma mou*. Chrisoula. *The golden one.*

I see your face light up when you open the door to your home, welcoming us in.

I imagine your hands, filling our plates with home-made chips. '*Faye, faye!* Eat, eat!'

I hear your laughter, tinkling, even in your darkest moments.

And your eyes. Your eyes. Kind, cheeky and wise. I look inside their blue depths, and they fill me with energy and love.

All I have to do is think of your voice, your touch, your gaze – through these you gave us so many golden gifts, *Mamma mou*. You showed us what it was like to feel welcome around a table. How to throw open one's doors, arms and heart to let people in. How to work hard for those you love. How to make things happen, gently but persistently, by being kind.

Twelve Golden Gifts

You have been giving me these gifts my whole life, even when I didn't realise it. Perhaps I didn't appreciate them enough in the past, but I know now how precious they are, how lucky I am to have them. I tried to use them as best I could to look after you in your time of greatest need.

I imagine you passing these gifts on to me. They are still warm with your touch. They sparkle with your intention, shine with your love and your golden spirit. I think of how I might put them to good use, as you have done so often in the past.

Once the gifts are in my hands, their golden energy flows through me, and words pour out and onto the page …

GIFT #1

Generosity

I will welcome you around my table

January 2020

Mum's hands are agitated, moving restlessly along the kitchen table, touching the stove that stands cold, switching the kettle on and off. She comes into the front room, where my brother Dennis and I are trying to set the large table. My children, Dolores and Emmanuel, are lying on the faded brown and tan velvet couch nearby, oblivious to anything their 81-year-old yiayia is doing. They are used to her fussing.

Mum repeats incessantly – *Do the kids want a drink? Do they want something to eat?* She laments that she hasn't cooked her usual *tyganites patates* – fried potatoes – and that the kids are going to *starve*.

'Mum, we're having fish and chips, remember? The whole point is that no one needs to cook. We can all relax.'

She nods, but looks a bit bereft.

Our first cousins, who we grew up with, are coming to visit. They now have adult children – and even a few grandchildren – of their own.

Mum hasn't contributed anything. Though she hasn't cooked for a large group since a stroke five years ago, she is unsettled. *It's not right. I should have cooked.* Her feeding impulse is like muscle memory – a lifetime of cooking for family and the many visitors that came to our home, isn't easily set aside.

Looking for ways to avert Mum's attention so we can set the table, I ask the kids to take her out to see what's growing in her garden. Mum's summer garden is a riot of lush tomatoes, cucumbers, basil and capsicums. She will watch proudly as Emmanuel scuttles in it to find the ripest tomatoes within the forest of vines. He will step onto the dark earth that she watered this morning, will come out bearing the bounty that she shares not just with us, but her sisters, my cousins and her neighbours. Though her kitchen is not operational today, her garden is still verdant with life.

*

After clearing the dining table of its embroidered tablecloth and oversized crystal vase, Dennis and I pull at its outer wings to extend it to its full seating capacity. Stiff with lack of use, we tease it upwards and outwards carefully before it gives. The seating won't be enough to accommodate our cousins and all their kids. The children will have to sit on the couch, plates on laps, just like we used to at large family gatherings.

While Dennis carefully sets out cutlery, plates and napkins, I look around the room. The thick lace curtains, which came with the house, are greying at the top. When my parents inspected the home 35 years ago, the real estate agent had the modest chandelier switched on, the light bouncing off an ornate built-in sideboard and mirror, highlighting the room's stuccoed solidity. This house was a big step up from the two-bedroom inner-city worker's cottage in Collingwood, the suburb we were living in at the time. Mum and Dad fretted about whether they could afford such a house. This stately front room no doubt clinched the deal.

The sideboard groans with photos of various weddings, my now-husband George and me cutting a cake at this very table at our engagement, and two statues of Greek goddesses. The drawers are filled with mismatched cutlery sets tied with cheap ribbon, the cupboards below with garishly coloured platters and dozens of demitasse coffee cups.

The last time all the coffee cups were pulled out of the sideboard was for my father's funeral wake, 15 years prior. The house and backyard were filled with people, dozens of garden chairs set out in every available space. My cousins and aunties ran around trying to serve Greek coffee and sweet rusks for a seemingly endless parade of family and friends. We'd agreed that when Mum died, we would have her wake catered for at the church hall. I make a mental note to sort through the sideboard's contents with Mum. Most of it will never get used again.

Dennis has finished setting up. His temples are greying, and his belly protrudes over the low belt of his pants. I recall a much darker-haired, thinner version of my brother, standing in this space 30 years ago on his 21st birthday. He'd not wanted a party, but my ever-social parents couldn't bear to let the occasion go unmarked. They would host a 'small' gathering of several dozen family friends and relatives. My cousin Jorge had organised a belly dancer. That night the floor shook with dancing bodies as she weaved her way around the guests. Several people pushed Dennis forward. He'd made an awkward-looking effort to swing his hips, click his fingers. When a burly uncle cut in, his hands much more eager to connect with the bejewelled hips of the dancer, Dennis's relief was palpable – he could retreat.

Dennis still lives with Mum, knows where everything is. We quickly finish the last of the preparations. For the past few years, our cousins and our family on my mother's side have been catching up annually each summer, often coinciding with Mum's birthday in January. As children we were in and out of each other's houses, but now it's quite the feat to organise a date where four generations might congregate.

The doorbell trills and the cousins and nieces and nephews arrive in a tsunami of colour and noise. Everyone smothers Mum with kisses, warm hugs. They place treats on the table – gifts of perfume, face creams and Greek cakes – all things they know Mum loves. Her face lights up, her agitation momentarily forgotten. Her joy at seeing loved ones at her door – my cousins are like her own children – is palpable.

Mum says it's too much; they shouldn't spend their money on her. That she prefers to give things, not the other way around.

'Nothing is too good for you, *Theia*, Aunty. You were our guardian angel growing up,' my first cousin Kathy enthuses. Kathy has a very special bond with Mum, fostered when our families spent a few years running a fish and chip shop in Narrandera in rural New South Wales during the '70s. I recall a pint-sized Kathy, sitting on the counter taking customer orders because she was too small to see over it, while Mum prepared the food behind her. As an adult, Mum and Dad looked after Kathy's daughter Sophia each day for two years while she worked. Now, Kathy delights in spoiling Mum: bringing her scratchies, watching her face light up as she rubs at them with a coin.

Dennis goes out to pick up the fish and chips, and when he returns, my cousin Dim divvies out food to the kids while her daughters pour soft drinks. Chaos reigns as we all speak over the top of each other. Drinks are spilled, sticky fingers wiped. Mum finally settles, allows her plate to be filled with food. She picks up a fork, looks up – *should she use it?*

'Just use your hands,' I tell her. There's no need for pretence here. She eats with gusto, as she has always done.

By the time we are finished, there are still piles of chips and dim sims on the table. As kids we would scrabble for the salty, crispy bits at the end, finish everything off. Then, it always felt as if there was never quite enough. Now we have too much.

When the table has been cleared, and the older kids gone for a walk with Uncle Dennis, the younger ones on the couch with their iPads, we settle into a post-lunch stupor. But Mum is agitated once again – she must make coffee to go with the sweets that my cousins have brought. Dim and I follow her into the kitchen and see her standing in front of the kettle, mug in hand. She looks confused, searches for the coffee, tries to pick up the spoon to stir the empty cup. Mum looks at us beseechingly.

'*Siga, siga*, Mum. Slowly, slowly,' I say. This was our refrain when she was recovering from the stroke several years ago that caused her problems such as recalling words and completing simple tasks. One word at a time. One task at a time. Within a year, she had made a surprising, if not complete, recovery.

'Now, let's turn the kettle on. Then we'll get the coffee …'

But her distress is obvious, and she can't still her mind long enough to go through each step. There are too many cups, too many people.

'We can make the coffees, Mum. How about you come inside and sit down?'

We take Mum back into the lounge. Dim looks concerned. She's a personal carer in a residential aged care home. It's clear she wants to say something.

Later, when we're washing the dishes in the kitchen, Dim says, 'I'm concerned about *Theia*. Vascular dementia is common in people who have had a stroke. Maybe you should get her tested.'

My knowledge of dementia is rudimentary at most. I know it's to do with the brain. That it affects memory and thinking, mood and behaviour. That it seems to happen mostly in older people.

If I could push back Dim's words, I would. I don't want to hear them. Mum has several friends in aged care homes who have dementia. Some are barely able to communicate, have withered away to a shadow of their former selves. When Mum and Dennis visit them, Mum often comes back flat. She's told me that having *anoia*, dementia, is one of her worst fears, that she would rather die than have it.

My initial defensiveness quickly morphs into the realisation that something crucial has changed. Recently, I have noticed Mum having lapses. She is starting to forget which ingredients go with which recipe. To forget in which drawer she might find her wooden spoon, where a particular pot lives. To forget that she needs to put carrots in a bean soup that she has been making since she was a child in Greece. She stands in her kitchen, midway between tasks, and wonders what she needs to do. It seems like a glitch, a hiccup in her thought process. She forces herself to stop, to take stock, to remember. When she can't, she stands there looking sad and lost.

I'm reminded of the early days after her stroke, when she had to teach herself to re-learn simple dishes, had to learn to pronounce words she had been using all her life, had to think carefully about each of the steps for daily tasks. It's like the clock is slowly turning back. My instinct to watch and see, to tread carefully, has stopped me from acting. But seeing her agitation, and Dim's words, make me think the time has come to explore what is going on.

Generosity

As the afternoon's festivities come to an end, Mum sees Dim off, tries to push money into her bag for the kids. There's a little tussle, and Dim quickly sidesteps her entreaties, waves goodbye. Is this beautiful generosity something that will eventually get lost? Will there come a time when she doesn't recognise us, when she can't tell us what she wants? And how to broach the sensitive topic of getting assessed for a condition that will ultimately lead to her demise? It's all too hard.

*

It's mid-April 2020 and we're having coffee at Mum's kitchen table. This table is smaller than the one in the front room but sees a lot more action: anytime someone drops in, biscuits from a well-worn Tupperware container are offered. If Mum is cooking, she will put out plates to share whatever is bubbling in her pot, sizzling in her frypan. Up until a few years ago, Mum was known for her ability to whip up *tyganopitara* (fried bread) and *loukoumathes* (honeyed donuts), comfort foods that could be prepared at the drop of a hat as soon as anyone stopped by. Flour and water, oil and sugar – simple ingredients, that in Mum's capable hands, helped bring a group of people around the table to talk and laugh.

A lot has happened in the past few months, including a little virus that's making its way around the world. The words 'global pandemic' are being touted. My husband George's father has had a serious fall and some concerning mental health episodes. There is talk of him going into residential aged care. Our whole family is now working and studying from home. Finding the right time to speak to Mum about seeing her doctor for a dementia diagnosis has been challenging.

Dennis has gone out for a walk. There's a box of *kourabiethes,* shortbreads dusted with icing sugar, between us. Mum pushes them towards me, urges me to take one.

Now's the time. I choose my words carefully.

'Mum, have things been harder lately, you know, with remembering things?'

'Yes, well, my words, since the stroke, I just can't talk, I can't remember the words …'

'I know. I see that sometimes you also have trouble in the kitchen, with remembering how to do things …'

'Yes. Yes.'

'Is it getting worse, do you think?'

She thinks about this, nods.

'Maybe we need to go to your doctor to find out what's going on?'

'If someone can help me with the words, it would be better …'

I've been holding my breath, anticipating her reaction. I let it go. She's willing to look into it. That's enough for now. I can get the ball rolling, make an appointment with her GP.

*

Generosity

The following week, her doctor, John, who she has been seeing since her stroke, greets her warmly in Greek, asks her how she is.

She starts with her customary refrain. 'Oh well, you know, I can't find my words …'

He smiles. 'I can understand you perfectly, *Kyria* Chrisoula.'

He does the usual checks – takes her blood pressure, listens to her heart, sees that she is up to date with her vaccinations. All the while I speak to him in English, knowing that Mum is unlikely to understand. Her English has always been limited, but since her stroke it has become even more so.

'Mum has been forgetting how to do basic things of late, like making a cup of coffee. And she seems to be having more trouble recalling words, like when she first had her stroke.'

He nods, doesn't miss a beat. Tells Mum he is going to ask her some questions in Greek.

'Now, there is no one to listen in, no journalists in the room, so you needn't worry about your performance.'

We all laugh. I get the impression John does this often.

'What year is it?'

Mum looks confused. She can't say.

'What season is it?' This she answers more confidently.

She's asked about what day it is, to repeat a set of items, to say where she is …

She gets some questions right, but there are quite a few she can't answer. She can't correctly copy a drawing. She starts to cry in frustration when she can't recall a series of words in the correct order. I can barely hold my own tears in, lean back a little to hide my face from her. Avert my eyes from John.

'It's alright, *Kyria* Chrisoula. You don't have to answer any more questions.'

'It's my words, they don't come …'

I'm not sure that I want to hear what John has to say. He turns to me.

'Look, likely she has trouble articulating the answers because of the stroke and the associated dysphasia …'

He checks to see if I am following. I nod. Since the stroke, Mum's ability to articulate the words she wants to say is impaired – there are times when she tries several times to find the right word. She can no longer read or write.

'But it's clear that there's more to it than that, that something else is going on. Let's start with blood tests and a CT head scan, and then we'll consider a referral to a memory clinic.' John explains to Mum in simple Greek what he is proposing, writes up the referrals.

Back at Mum's house, we sit at the kitchen table and mull over what might be happening. She cries some more. I try to reassure her, say it's important to work out what's going on so we can help her. I keep my voice light and hopeful, trying to convince myself too. But though her language and memory might be impaired, she's no fool. She's had a lifetime of adversity – born during wartime, surviving a depression, marrying and raising kids in a foreign country, working long days in a manual job and nursing her husband through a cruel disease that took him too early. She's got enough life experience to know that whatever is going on now, it can't be good.

When it's time for me to go home, she takes charge once again, bringing out the organic eggs that she buys from a farmer who delivers them to her home.

'These are fresh. No chemicals. Take this milk too. Emmanuel is growing. Feed him as much as you can!'

As always, it comes back to the language of food, of love. In this she is well versed.

*

A few weeks later, when I get to Mum's house, she is waiting at the front door – bag on her shoulder, neatly dressed in dark satin blouse and blue skirt, stockings and shiny shoes with a wedge heel.

I hesitate before giving her a kiss – is it safe? We have been in a city-wide lockdown for the past few months due to the risk of contracting Covid. The only reason I can be here is that I have a carer's letter from her doctor. But virus or no virus, a lifetime of habit is hard to break. We kiss on both cheeks. Dennis hovers nearby. He's never been comfortable with bodily contact, and the threat of a sinister virus is a good excuse to dispense with kisses.

Mum's bag doesn't hold much but her purse and a clean hanky. I double check that she has her Medicare and pension cards. Her purse bulges with coins that she collects for church, and a crisp $100 note.

'You don't need that much money, Mum.'

'We might have to pay for the test.'

'I'm pretty sure Medicare will pay for it.' I don't say that if it isn't bulkbilled, it's likely to be more than $100. 'I can always pay for it on my card.'

'Doesn't matter. You should never leave the house without money.'

This makes me smile. My father would also say this. When you walked out of your home, you had to be prepared for all contingencies. Cash could get you out of all sorts of mischief.

I fossick through the detritus in my own bag, take out the referral for the CT head scan. The radiology clinic is just up the road from Mum's. We're still early, but she wants to get going.

When we get to the clinic, the car park is empty. As we round the corner, we see that the doors are closed and locked. There's a sign on the door indicating that the service has been shut due to Covid-19. After making a harried call, I'm told she can be seen at their Richmond facility, a suburb some 20 minutes away. It's at the city end of Bridge Road, a strip with which I'm familiar. We get back into the car.

Mum sits forward in her seat, agitated. 'I'm putting you out. Why are we even having this test anyway?'

'Because the doctor just wants to see why you have been forgetting. I'm happy to take you, Mum.' I quickly change the subject. 'Remember when we used to come to the market around here?'

She looks out the window, nods hesitantly.

As a teenager, our family would shop at a fresh food market on one of these Richmond streets, which was closed off for the purpose each Saturday morning. We would make our way past each stall, looking to see who had the cheapest, freshest produce. The pace became frenzied at closing time as vendors competed to get rid of everything, calling out prices and waving their arms wildly in a bid to attract customers. Boxes of overripe and blemished produce that hadn't quite passed muster earlier would lay at their feet. This was Mum's opportunity to buy up big. It wasn't unusual to take a whole box of fruit home and eat it all at once before it went off.

While Mum was scooping up the specials, Dad was more discerning. He would carefully inspect the fish available at one stall, choosing a whole snapper or bream, perhaps some sardines. Mum would clean these when we got home and bake or fry them. Occasionally, I would get a jam donut from a nearby van. My parents and I would then lug our trolley and any boxes to the car several streets away.

The market still runs, but now it sells sourdough bread, handmade pastries, organic coffee. The sturdy-looking Italians who ran the show back in the day have been replaced by boutique farmers and artisanal provedores.

Further down Bridge Road, we drive past boutiques that were once bustling with activity. When I was a teenager, Mum and I would come here to fossick through chaotic racks of samples and slightly shop-soiled dresses at a fraction of the cost of what one might pay in the department stores and boutiques in the city. She would wait patiently while I tried things on, rarely buying anything for herself. Even during my sulky teen years, I always respected her opinion.

Now, it seems as if every second shop sports a 'For Lease' sign. It's likely been years in the making as the oversized outlets peppered around Melbourne have seduced customers away from the inner suburbs. Online shopping, and now the lockdowns, are probably the nails in the coffin. Seeing the empty shopfronts saddens me – it's like a part of my history is gone.

We finally get to the clinic, set along a blue-stone cobbled lane. It's one of various medical businesses that nudges up to apartments and terrace houses that have been extended and renovated, a Tetris of buildings that have been packed into every available space. I take Mum's arm so that she doesn't trip on the uneven ground.

We take a seat inside and let the receptionist know we are here. We are given a form to fill in with Mum's details and medical history, which I complete for her as I have done from the time I learnt to write. We need to sanitise our hands. There's tape on the floor, indicating we must stand 1.5 metres away from the staff and each other. It feels surreal, as if we are on the set of a science-fiction movie. Is all this necessary? I lean my head in to talk quietly with Mum. She repeats that it's all too much trouble. That I need to be working. That my family needs me.

'Mum, please don't worry. Work is never ending – it will be there for me to do tomorrow. And the kids are older now – they are fine. I like being with you.'

Spending time with Mum, albeit waiting for a CT scan, is a welcome relief from routine. Mum settles, eyeballs a woman wearing garish Lycra pants that stretch thin over her generous bottom. Mum looks at me. We don't need to speak. She starts to giggle. I nudge her to stop. But soon her contagious laugh has me going too.

I force myself to settle down. 'You used to take time off work so we could shop together, even though you were busy sewing. Remember how you used to get up so early, and not go to bed until late at night?' I say.

She nods. How could she forget her nearly 50-year history of sewing. There was always a tower of nighties on her overlocking machine. I recall the swift movement of her strong fleshy arms as she picked up two pieces, lined them up; and the thin film of cotton dust as she ran them through the machine.

One memory leads to another. 'Do you remember Dimmeys, Mum?'

She smiles at the memory of the discount emporium, which sold everything from dress lining to linen, drapes to door stops. We spent many an afternoon walking through upright rolls of fabric; fossicking through a chaotic array of bargain bins filled with fabric offcuts and discounted clothes. There were buttons displayed in plastic tubes, countless spools of coloured thread, sewing needles in all shapes and sizes, and oversized books of patterns. Mum and I would pore over these whenever we had a formal occasion coming up, and I would point out a style I'd like her to replicate. We'd spend hours choosing the right fabric, buttons and zips. Invariably, she would make her own patterns, and I would sit with her, doing simple stitching, or sewing on buttons. Watching her work was a joy – one of the rare occasions when I felt I had her all to myself.

'It's all in the finishes, Spiridoula,' she would say. 'Neat buttonholes, lovely buttons, and then the final press with the iron. Even if you are poor and can't afford expensive fabrics, you can still look good. In Greece, most people could only afford a new outfit for Easter. If they were lucky ...'

Her eyes would get that far away, sad look. Thinking about her homeland always made her wistful.

'Do you still use the sewing machines?' Mum has two industrial sewing machines in her garden bungalow.

'Just to take up pants ... I find the overlocker hard to thread.'

She used to be able to do it without thinking. Dennis has been searching on YouTube to help her. I sigh. Another skill lost.

We are called up and led to a small cubicle. I translate the instructions. *Remove any jewellery and metal objects. Take off the top half of your clothes, including bra, and place them in a basket, put the gown on.* When she comes out, the ties on the back of the garment are hanging. I notice the freckles on her back, cover her up protectively. She removes her lower denture, as it has a metal bit, and places it into the hanky from her bag. Her lower lip caves inwards and she looks older, somehow smaller. She is not as plump as she used to be.

We walk to a room where she is told to lie very still on a bed below a circle-shaped scanner. I help her up. I'm asked to leave the room, but hang by the door. What if she needs me to explain something? She looks so vulnerable on the hard bed. But the radiologist assures me he will call me if I'm needed. Ten minutes later, she comes out.

'Everything okay?'

'Yes, yes. Now, hurry up so we can go home. It's time to eat.' She's preparing fried artichokes and eggs, which she knows is one of my favourite dishes.

She fossicks in her bag for her dentures and slips them in. Her face is once again her own. She no longer looks so vulnerable. She has cooking to do. I slip my arm into hers, and we head home.

*

We follow up the CT scan with another visit to her doctor, John. He pulls up the scan results.

'I can see damage from the stroke, but there's not much evidence of other damage. And the blood tests are normal. That doesn't mean there's nothing going on. It might be a while before you can get an appointment, but I can refer you to a memory clinic.'

'What are the benefits of getting a formal diagnosis ... say, if it is some sort of dementia?'

'Well to be frank, in your Mum's case there might not be many options for medication to slow the disease down. But a diagnosis could help with her care down the track.'

John's mother lives in the same suburb as Mum, goes to the same church. Mum often asks after her.

'If it was your Mum, would you send her?'

He pauses for a moment. 'Yes, yes I would.'

We walk out with a referral for the memory clinic.

*

It's autumn, and we are in the thick of a lockdown. This was unthinkable months ago. I go for a walk to take a break from the monotony of talking at pixelated icons, droning on and on, sick of myself and my inability to impart anything meaningful to the writing students I teach, whose eyes and body language I can't see. They drop away like flies as the weeks go on.

George, who's in the middle of a virtual meeting at the kitchen table, waves goodbye. Dolores looks up from her laptop in the loungeroom and goes back to listening to her lecture. Emmanuel is in his room, door closed. He too is having an online class. His final year at high school is being taught via a screen, but he doesn't seem too fussed. It's working for him.

I leave it all behind me and make my daily phone call to Mum.

'How are you, Mum?'

'Good, good. When are you coming?'

'Friday. In two days. What did you have for lunch?'

Hearing Mum's voice, talking about her routines – watering her garden, walking around the block, having lunch with Dennis – is reassuring. Not much has changed for her since the lockdowns, except that she isn't seeing as many people and is not going to church. It's been hard to explain what the virus is all about, why people can't visit like they used to. I'm lucky, I can still see her to give Dennis help with her care, and to get my fill of her. I ask her what she would like me to bring on Friday, and she says, '*Tipota. Esei ftaneis.*' Nothing. You're enough.

After I've hung up, I see a father playing footy on the street with his young son – the lockdown has at least given them this time together. My mother always sees the silver lining, and I have inherited her optimism. At least we are all safe. Our family is spending time together that we wouldn't normally have. Thank goodness we don't have young kids who need to be homeschooled. We still have jobs, a home large enough that we can move in and out of each other's space. We're like the valve of a beating heart, coping by making each other endless cups of tea, sitting together each day around the table or television. George has been baking bread, tending to the garden. I go on daily walks between classes, ring an elderly uncle or my cousins. It's not so bad.

On the bush path near our home there are dogs – so many dogs. There are also families out with their bikes, couples walking, singles jogging. I think about Mum again and this time tears threaten. It's been a long time since I've cried, but these past few days, it's all I've been doing. Tears come at random, inconvenient moments, and I don't trust myself to hold them in. The decision to have Mum assessed has sparked something in me – I think I already know what the outcome is going to be.

I'd made the call to the memory clinic – they were not making in-person appointments because of the lockdowns. They'd asked whether Mum would like an online appointment with an interpreter. I don't think this will work given Mum's communication issues and ask to be put on a waiting list for when the service re-opens.

I'm still not sure about whether a diagnosis of dementia will help Mum, whether it might throw her into despair. Her quality of life is good. She still speaks with both her sisters each day. She still manages to cook simple meals. She can still clean her house, though this has become harder, slower. She does not appear to be depressed.

But if I'm honest with myself, the glitches are getting worse. She seems to be getting frailer. She appears more confused, more often. She is more agitated, is unable to sit still for any length of time. She goes into overdrive with giving things away, giving the kids money, plying me with food. She repeats herself obsessively.

As I walk, I think about the pumpkin sitting on the bench at home, the one my husband grew. I know now how to deal with these tears, this sadness, at least for today. I will cook. I will cook pumpkin soup.

Mum taught me to cook. She was patient with me. She didn't carry on if I didn't get it right. Rather, she cleverly complimented me on what I did well, then gently suggested what I might do better. She gifted me a lifelong love of the kitchen as a place to bring people together, to nurture them, to give them pleasure and sustenance.

When I get home, I will cleave the pumpkin, denuding it of its seeds and pale skin. There will be the satisfying wet sound of firm flesh yielding to the knife. I will put the cut-up pumpkin in a tray, with garlic and rosemary, along with the stock left over from a lamb roast. I love that a few bones that would otherwise be thrown away still have something to give; how one meal can contribute to another – why throw something away when it still has flavour in it? This is also Mum's doing – for she taught me to be frugal.

As I walk, contemplating what lies ahead, I worry that soon Mum may not be able to walk unattended around her neighbourhood, may not be able to be unsupervised around a stove or in the shower. I hope it takes years, not months.

I jump ahead, imagine my life without her, and the tears start once more.

I pull myself up. I think of all the times that Mum delivered soup to me when my children were young – how comforting it was. I think about making her pumpkin soup. Delivering it with fresh bread. We will sit together around her table to eat. The image is energising. I hurry back home.

GIFT #2

Openness

I will greet you at my door with open arms and heart

July 2020

It's now mid-winter and the weeks of elastic-waisted pants and predictable routines seem endless: waking up, downing coffee, sweeping the floor, tidying up; making my way out to our garden studio to teach and trying to work out how to retain our students, coming back inside to share lunch or cups of tea with the other homebound members of the family; walking around the same blocks for my daily exercise and coming in to cook, have dinner, watch television and drink too much wine; waking the next morning to do it all again. The early weeks of enthusiastic baking are behind us. The easing and tightening, easing and tightening of restrictions is disconcerting, the goal posts constantly changing. We are now back in a lockdown. When will it be over?

It's clear we aren't the only ones keen to see the back of the lockdowns. I get a call from the memory clinic. The worker there tells me they are struggling to see the many people on their waiting list due to the lockdowns. She has Mum's results, notes that Mum has a clear head scan and nebulous symptoms. As a fellow Greek speaker, she hints that Greek women of Mum's generation find the process of diagnosis quite onerous – they must answer lots of questions, do lots of tests.

'Perhaps Chrisoula doesn't need an appointment anymore?' she asks hopefully.

I imagine the long list of people waiting for the precious appointments, and her relief at being able to take a name off her list. But I've got to do what's best for Mum. I tell her I will think about it, will ring her back.

Her comments spark my doubt about whether it's in Mum's best interests to get a diagnosis. To help me decide, I make a flurry of calls.

First, I ring Dementia Australia. They tell me that there are many support services available for people with dementia and their carers. While there is a lot of free information, some of the services available can only be accessed after a diagnosis.

Next, I speak with our family friend Tina, whose mother Efrosini has dementia, and who now lives with her. Tina says that a formal diagnosis helped her organise services for her mother through My Aged Care, the government body that subsidises in-home and residential care services. These help fund transport to and from social activities for her Mum a few times each week. This has made a big difference to her Mum's wellbeing. It's also reassuring for Tina, who works full time, knowing her Mum is occupied and safe.

Tina also tells me about enduring power of attorney. She explains that we can make some decisions on Mum's behalf when she can no longer make these decisions herself. Though my brother and I have been managing Mum's finances and correspondence since her stroke, Tina encourages me to formalise the process before Mum declines further and isn't fit to decide. I bookmark the forms on the Office of the Public Advocate website, add them to the list of things to get my head around. I am not sure how Mum will feel about this, and have to think about how to broach it with her.

What this research makes me realise is that it will help Mum to get diagnosed, if only to give her access to services down the track when her condition worsens. I ring the memory clinic back, make an appointment.

*

We convene for dinner each night. It's a ritual both George's and my family imparted to us growing up, and it's one that we try to uphold with my own family whenever possible. But conversations about our elderly parents hang like a cloud over this formerly joyful ritual. I feel for Dolores and Emmanuel as they listen silently, their faces grim.

George's dad has been newly admitted to an aged care home. Visits are conducted with George standing in the home's yard, talking to his distressed father through a window in 15-minute increments, watching him hobble away on his walker. There are other visitors lined up behind him, eager to have their turn. His mother is alone in the family home. In 60 years of marriage, she hasn't spent more than a night away from my father-in-law. George and his sister are sharing the burden of staying with her overnight while she adjusts. Inevitably George feels flat after these visits, guilty and desperately needing to offload. He says that admitting his father into an aged care home during lockdowns was the saddest day of his life.

The visits to Mum's house are now much more regular. I visit her every Friday, and other days requiring medical appointments – we have a heady cocktail of these lined up – x-rays, vaccinations, blood tests. Dennis often uses the time to go out for a walk or to shop.

I get into pants that aren't bound by elastic, put on a colourful top, a peel of red lipstick; start to look something like my former self, even if the band on my pants is getting too tight for my expanding belly. I shop for ingredients I know Mum will love – salmon fillets, a piece of premium steak, oodles of colourful vegetables to be pan fried until their colours come alive with garlic, olive oil and heat.

Mum's face lights up when she sees me at her doorstep.

'Come in, come in!' Her sense of joy at seeing me is palpable. No matter what is going on, I am always welcome with open arms at her doorstep. I appreciate this more than ever during this difficult time. The grim cloud that hangs over our own dinner table fades away when I am here.

I try to resist the urge to lean in for a hug or kiss. Mum tells me off for bringing food, even as she looks in the bags to see what I've bought. Her simple joy at eating a delicious meal is infectious. My brother and I bash around, looking for the right pots. Mum comes in and out of the kitchen, looking for ways to be helpful. I ask her for herbs from her garden, things I know she can help with. We set the table with a worn Australiana tablecloth from the '70s, place each dish in the middle of the table to be shared, the traditional way of eating in Greece.

I watch as Mum tucks into the dish with gusto, always leaving the tastiest morsel until last. She always ate fast, said it was a sign of being *prokommeni,* capable and efficient. And she's always enjoyed her food.

She teases me about not using enough salt, for being too conservative with the oil. My aunty sends us vats of oil from Greece. Mum often comes up behind me when I'm cooking and adds more. The banter, the simple joy of creating a meal, and eating it together, is energising for all of us. When we're finished, Dennis washes the dishes while Mum and I go for a walk around the block.

Mum calls out to *Kyria* Eleni, a Cypriot neighbour, who is sitting on the porch with her daughter-in-law and grandchild. She manages to convey to me that *Kyria* Eleni's father went to Cyprus for a holiday and was unable to return because of the pandemic. Mum says hello to an Italian woman who greets her warmly. Mum's eyes twinkle as she makes herself perfectly understood, even with the limited English words available to her. She crosses the road to avoid the dog that barks too loudly. She looks for oncoming traffic when she steps off the curb. I have become apprehensive about her getting lost, perhaps being run over, as a local Greek woman was some years prior. But her gait is considered. She carefully steps over the dips and cracks in the footpath, doesn't stray from the loop that is the big block around her house; and a surprising number of people know her. If she were to get lost, someone she knows would likely walk her home. Taking away the freedom of going for a walk on her own anytime she likes feels a little premature. And so, I start to relax, let her knowledge of these streets, and the people in them, wash over me. I loop my arm through hers.

'That's *Kyria* Tasia's house. New people have bought it. And that's where *Kyria* Sophia used to live. They're both dead now. *Achh* …'

We walk past so many houses where Greek-speaking neighbours lived, and who have now died. Their legacy lives on in the fruit trees they planted in their front yards, in the fake-brick cladding they put up to avoid painting weatherboards, in the fences that have outlived them. Mum notes how quickly time has passed since we moved here with our family in 1985, when the suburb was filled with young families. Her stories are peppered with sadness as she tries to find the words, recall the names of each person who lived here, the connections between them. Regularly, obsessively, she laments how her stroke has robbed her of words. I counter with reassurances on repeat. *I understand it's not easy. Take it slowly. Most people you speak to understand you.* But it's becoming more than that – even when she remembers the words, can string them together, she soon forgets them again. They slip in and out of her head, elusive. For someone whose greatest strength was her ability to speak, to communicate, it must be so frustrating. And depressing. But I watch as she connects with the people on her walk, am surprised by how many people know her by first name. I am, yet again, in awe of my mother.

'I could die tomorrow you know. It would be better that way. I wouldn't trouble anyone. I've lived my life,' she says.

'Yes. But you can't control when you'll die, Mum. It doesn't always happen easily ...'

I think about Dad, who spent the final months of his life in a hospital bed with motor neurone disease. I remember a skeletal leg poking out from under the sheet in the last weeks before he died. The family meeting where doctors broke the news to him that his condition was terminal. Mum angry at me because I'd insisted that this was information he needed to know.

Mum nods. She has enough life experience to know that dying isn't always easy.

'Anyway, you might be ready, but I'm not!' I say. I try to keep my tone light.

'I don't want you crying when I'm dead. And don't spend money on a wake. Just keep living your life.'

'Mum, as if I wouldn't cry for you. And you've fed so many people. Of course we're going to have a wake. With lots of food!'

We keep walking silently, each in our own thoughts. Thinking of Mum dying makes me tear up. I think of the prayer 'Grant me the serenity to accept the things I cannot change, the courage to change the things I can, and the wisdom to know the difference.' I'm sure there's a 'God' in there somewhere. I wish I had Mum's unshakeable belief in a higher power, her faithful dedication to her religion that plays out in the daily lighting of her *kandili*, a vigil candle, and regular churchgoing. I envy her that certainty, that reassurance. For me, there would just be a gaping hole where my once robust Mum stood. I clutch at her elbow more securely, force myself to come back to the present.

When we return to her home, Mum is all anxious activity just in case she should forget something. She pulls two three-litre cartons of milk out of the fridge, places several bottles of laundry liquid and packets of toilet paper onto the kitchen table, sneaks an envelope of money for the children into my bag. There is a tussle to resist this – *Mum, we buy these things ourselves, you don't need to get them for us* – but as always, she wins the battle. As I head off, she stands on the porch in front of her open door and doesn't go back in until I have safely turned the corner. Not for the first time, I wonder: who is caring for whom?

*

I'm not looking forward to the delicate conversation with Mum about enduring power of attorney.

Dennis and I have been signatories to Mum's bank account for several years. We manage and pay her bills, organise and accompany her to appointments with health providers. We are already very involved in her affairs, but this is taking the next big leap. It won't be an easy talk to have, and I feel the need to tread carefully.

When next at Mum's, I explain the process as I understand it: that we will always speak with her and ask her how she wants to manage things as we have always done – but if she finds one day she can't manage, we will be able to make decisions for her. That it is good for us to have these chats now, so she can tell us what she would like. What should we do if she was to have another stroke, if she became unconscious for example, would she like to be revived?

'Just let me die. I don't want to live like that!'

I go on, explain that we would have the power to sell her house if we needed to, to pay for care. I want to make it clear in a very practical way what she would be agreeing to in the worst-case scenario.

'I'm not going to a nursing home. I want to die here!'

'Yes, I know, Mum. But this is just *if* it should happen.'

'Well, I don't want you to sell the house. After I die, you can knock it down. Build two houses. Live next to each other. And *don't fight!*'

Openness

I sigh. Her concern about what will happen to Dennis after she dies has been a recurring worry over the years. As always, she prioritised looking after us rather than herself.

Mum has always been very protective over Dennis, who has lived with her his whole life. She's always cared for him, but since her stroke, the tables have turned, with Dennis stepping up considerably to support Mum. It hasn't been easy, but they've managed to make it work. If it wasn't for Dennis, Mum would unlikely still be living at home.

It's not the first time she's spoken about Dennis and me living next to each other, about her wanting us to continue having an amicable relationship. And about what she wants us to do with her home, which she has worked so hard for. I think she imagines me walking food over to Dennis, him coming over to watch TV with our family. It's a nice fantasy, but we already have a house, one that we have spent a lot of energy into making a home. And I don't think Dennis would be wanting to live in such close proximity to us either.

'Don't worry, Mum. Dennis and I won't fight. I promise.'

We talk some more about the power of attorney process. I feel confident she understands what I am saying. What she is agreeing to is no small thing, but she is a bit confused about why it's needed.

'Hopefully we will never need to step in. But it makes it easier if we must. And it's better to do it now.' I pause, let the unspoken words lie between us. *If you no longer have the cognition, and the words, to say what you want.*

'Do you trust us, Mum?' I ask.

She looks at Dennis and me, and nods. 'Yes.'

I explain that we will need to complete some forms, that likely we will meet with her doctor or a lawyer to talk her through what she is agreeing to and sign them. I promise to find out more, will let her know what she needs to do. She gives me permission to go ahead. Not for the first time, I'm grateful to Mum for being so open to talking about difficult things. Dad, who avoided talking about death or wills at all costs, went to his grave without a will. A few short weeks later, Mum had me organise the lawyer to draw up a will. She wanted to have her affairs in order.

Still, once these forms are done, I hope we never have to refer to them again.

*

I download and start to complete the enduring power of attorney documents from the Office of the Public Advocate: one for appointing a medical treatment decision-maker, and another for making personal and financial decisions on Mum's behalf. On opening the forms, I realise there are some things I don't understand. If we have two attorneys, how can they act together? Is it okay for Mum's doctor to sign the forms, or do we need to go through a solicitor?

An operator at the Office of the Public Advocate answers my questions. She pointedly states that Mum's best interests need to be protected, reiterates the need for Mum to understand and agree to this process, that due diligence needs to be followed. I can see why she would be concerned: elder abuse is all too common. I can also see how our having so much power over Mum's affairs might be abused, yet part of me rankles. *We would never abuse Mum's interests.* But she doesn't know us, and she's just doing her job, which I can appreciate isn't an easy one.

She explains that we can fill out the forms ourselves with Mum's input, and get her doctor to sign them, or we can go through a solicitor to get them completed. One of the forms numbers nearly 30 pages. As Dennis and I are both signatories, I will need to speak with him about how we will act together, and state this clearly on the form. I then need to make a time with Mum's doctor to sign them when Mum can be present. I thank her for her time, make an appointment with Mum's GP, and turn back to my computer to complete as much of the form as I can.

*

With the enduring power of attorney completed, and a visit to Mum's doctor to sign the forms, I can now turn to more practical matters: a bit of decluttering to help Mum navigate her home more easily.

The idea is to help her cull a lifetime's worth of linen, towels, clothes, shoes and other miscellany, a task she is no longer able to manage herself. It's early on a Saturday morning, and I've left my own house in a mess, my teens still sleeping, my husband tending our garden.

I'm not far in when I find a jewellery box at the top of a wardrobe. When I take it down, it feels lighter, less substantial than I remember it. Its surface is dull where once it gleamed with the weekly spray of Mr Sheen. Its Japanese design was popular in the '70s. Hand-painted mountain peaks and traditional Minka houses decorate its lacquered top and sides. It used to have pride of place on Mum's baroque-style vanity. As a young child, I never tired of watching the ballerina that spun every time you opened the lid, her pale pink tutu and golden head of hair turning slowly as a tinny tune played until you slid the lid back down.

The jewellery box was filled with glittering treasure brought back from the old country: a thick, ornate bangle with an intriguingly complicated clasp; two British sovereigns bequeathed by my grandfather; gold crosses and tiny bracelets given by our godparents at Dennis's and my christenings, cushioned in padded boxes with the names of Greek jewellers written in gilt on their lids; and a diamond-shaped pendant that would nestle in Mum's bosom when she wore it on very special occasions.

It takes all my willpower to stop myself from looking inside. To do that will take me down the cobbled road of the past, dragging me away from what needs to be done. I cannot, *will not*, be distracted.

Back on the stepladder, I pull down a cardboard box, tied tightly with twine. This cuts into my fingers and I struggle to ease it off, but finally the lid pops open to reveal baby clothes. I lift several dresses my mother-in-law brought back from Malta; dresses that once belonged to my sister-in-law, also worn by my daughter when she was a baby. These are snuggled alongside tiny handknitted booties and little jackets with satin ties that my in-laws arranged to have knitted before our children were born, presenting them to us in the suitcase they came to Australia with. There are woollen bonnets and bodysuits that make me laugh when I think that the bodies they once clothed now tower over me. I *coo* and *ahh*, but quickly make myself place the items back in the box, pushing the flaps back down. *I will not be distracted.*

It's not long after that I come across a vinyl sleeve with faded red roses and a gold border; I'm guessing a make-up bag from the '70s. I open the flap to reveal photos: dozens upon dozens of images of weddings in front of white churches and people standing in mud-streaked village fields; snaps of women in minidresses posing in hallways, and babies being baptised in burnished metal basins.

These are photos Mum lent me several years ago when I wrote a memoir and needed prompting to tell my story and that of my family. The photos had gone missing, and I feared I'd lost them in the detritus of my own home. Every now and then Mum and I would talk about them. She insisted I still had them, but I could only find a handful in my study.

I call out to Mum, 'I've found the photos! I've found them.'

I take the sleeve out to the loungeroom and place it carefully on the coffee table. Mum joins me. She smiles sadly.

'We keep. To remember,' she says in Greek. Since the stroke some years ago, even her Greek is garbled, but there is no mistaking the sentiment.

'Yes, to remember.' I try to ignore the pangs of sadness that threaten to simmer to the surface; am reminded yet again more time has elapsed in both our lives than lies ahead. These pangs seem to appear with alarming regularity these days: when Mum tells me of yet another friend or family member dying; when my husband and I grunt with the effort of bending to pick something up; seeing our daughter and her friend off on an interstate trip without us …

I pull out one of the photos, revealing a pale, shy-looking woman clad head to toe in voile and lace; a skinny, dark-skinned man beside her. This pair is flanked by a handsome couple, who look worldlier, more knowing. I know the bride and groom are my parents, but looking at my mother beside me now, you wouldn't recognise her as the young woman in the photo. Her skin is wrinkled and her body stooped; her movements are tentative, as if she has forgotten how to be in her own home, much less outside of it. But as I look into her eyes, I still see something of the spirit of that new bride in a new country with no English and no money, getting married to a man she barely knew. A woman who was forced to look forward, not back, in

Openness

a bid to survive. That young woman is still in there, and her playful eyes tell me she has wised up a lot since then.

I pull myself out of my reverie. This is something to savour later. I carefully place the photos back down on the coffee table and return to the wardrobe.

Thankfully the task becomes easier as the treasures become more mundane – piles of linen, towers of blankets and comforters, mounds of shoes. We get to work in earnest: sort and place their contents in neat piles; designate a space for things that belong to the op shop; another for things that need to be binned; yet another for stuff that needs Mum's input. Dennis helps take piles away, vacuums dusty corners, advises about things that are his.

Mum potters around us, trying to be helpful. It becomes apparent that there are piles hidden away in every corner, and that even she doesn't know what she has. Mum seems to have a fetish for linen, with drawers and cupboards filled with doilies, tablecloths, doonas and sheet sets. There are cupboards full of platters and crystal glasses gifted during the many parties that my parents hosted over the years, radios and stereos that haven't properly worked for decades, VHS tapes with footage from naming days and weddings, cassette tapes with Greek blues from the '50s, drawers full of photo albums and enough photo frames to fill a small gallery. What was to be a quick clean-up turns into a prolonged ordeal.

As I'm stripping and culling, casting and curbing, I see shades of my parents' and our lives reflected in every object, in every dusty corner and packed wardrobe. The feelings this exercise dredges up threaten to overwhelm me. After my Mum is gone, we will have to clear even more of her home. What will remain of her but a few choice objects and memories of who she was and how she made us feel? Is this what a life comes down to anyway?

As I've gotten older, I've come to see the appeal of combing over memories again and again, picking them up and turning them over this way and that so as to remind ourselves that the life we have lived means something. That it's not just about the big milestones – births and christenings, weddings and birthdays – but the small pivotal moments.

What happens when you no longer remember? When the memories disappear? Does this mean you, as you know yourself and all your collective experiences, cease to exist?

I reflect that it's reassuring to think that we continue to live in the experiences and thoughts of others.

Mum has a wardrobe packed with formal clothes. It includes shirts and jackets, skirts and pants, most of which she made herself and rarely wears. Now, when she needs to go out, she spends a long time looking for a skirt that still fits, a jacket that she doesn't swim in.

Mum sits down on the bed, and I hold each piece of clothing for her to look at. What becomes clear is that most outfits are two or three sizes too big for her. After Mum's initial hesitation and sadness at the many memories attached to the clothes she carefully made to wear to important family events, she becomes practical: if I tell her it's too big, she lets me place it in the pile destined for the op shop. Items she wears regularly are placed neatly in the drawers in her room.

Mum has already told me that she wants to wear the gold dress she wore to my wedding at her funeral. She points it out, makes sure I know which one it is. I don't dare tell her that it may be way too big now she has lost so much weight. There are some silky undergarments packed in a plastic bag at the top of her wardrobe that she would also like to wear – she's thought of everything. Finally, she reminds me about the shoes – *don't forget the shoes!* She doesn't want to be treading the pathway up to heaven in bare feet.

In the afternoon, Mum potters around the house doing small, manageable tasks, advises when asked, agrees with most of the decisions made. I'm pleased that we are doing this now, not when she is gone.

It feels satisfying to cull things in order to let spaces breathe, to get rid of the physical stuff that so often weighs one down. For Mum, it's yet another thing completed as she nears the end of her life, along with paying for her gravestone and choosing which outfit she wants to be buried in.

She's always taken pride in keeping a tidy house, cleaning regularly. It feels good to be able to help her get her house back into a semblance of order. After a while, we become efficient and ruthless – do we keep, gift or throw away? I ask Mum repeatedly: When was the last time you used this? How many sheet sets do you *really* need anyway?

Some hours later, several large bags sit beside the rubbish bin for disposal. A carload of items has been delivered to the op shop. The baby clothes have been labelled and placed back into the wardrobe to look at again when we next visit Mum with our kids. The only thing left on Mum's bed is the jewellery box. Seeing it there dredges up memories long forgotten. Mum and Dad would regularly check its contents to see that everything was in its place, the provenance of each piece spoken about reverently. Its very existence was proof that my parents had raised themselves out of the poverty of their rural Greek roots. Along with their single-fronted worker's cottage, and the small amounts of cash they could save from their factory jobs, the treasures within were insurance in case they should ever face such poverty again.

Not a little apprehensively, I open the lid of the box and the first thing I notice is the absence of music. The ballerina isn't spinning. Her dress is faded. She leans a little to one side, perhaps because of my overzealous attentions all that time ago. Her golden locks are simply a lick of paint. The box is strangely bare, with dust and grime clinging to its velveteen lining. It holds a filigreed gold brooch, a few worn and mismatched earrings, the box's tiny key and a small envelope. Inexplicably, it also houses two digital thermometers. I wonder what happened to the jewels, must ask Mum later, see if her answer makes sense.

She may not be able to convey it, even if she does remember. Like the questions about the family tree I had kept meaning to ask her, maybe it's too late.

I open the envelope and see several gold caps, some with teeth still attached. With a dawning sense of horror, I realise they belonged to my father. Perhaps they were removed after he died. I have a sudden and sickening vision of teeth being pulled from my father's flesh by an anonymous undertaker as he prepared his body for the viewing at the funeral. But the answer is probably more prosaic – more likely he had them removed when he got dentures several years prior to his dying. And no doubt the gold was too precious to throw away.

Mum comes into the room and finds me crumpling the envelope in my hand. She looks into my eyes, looks at my hands. She hesitates, but there's no getting away from the question that must come next.

'What's in there?'

I too hesitate. We've done so well up until now.

'Dad's gold teeth.'

A pained, sad look comes over her, all too familiar these days as she laments the losses that have appeared like cracks since her stroke. We both tear up.

'Throw them away,' she says.

'I don't want to. They're part of him.'

There is a moment of mutual understanding. She looks down at the open jewellery box, glances at its meagre contents briefly.

'Take it then. I don't need it anymore.'

'Are you sure?'

She nods. She's sure. This feels like another letting go of things that are no longer important, physical things that she won't be able to take with her when she goes.

And so, the jewellery box is added to the other things I am taking away with me: a box of brand-new towels we bought her a few Christmases ago, two transistor radios our son is going to love; several Greek books she can no longer read that I might flick through before adding to our own overwhelming piles of books.

It's late afternoon and the time has come to go home to my family. I silently commend myself on a great day's work, cast one look at the wardrobe as I prepare to leave. Everything is placed neatly, with Mum's personal things within easy reach for her. The only thing still left out is the sleeve filled with photos. These we will have to deal with on another day.

*

We're sitting at Mum's kitchen table. I'm doing a sales pitch, telling her that the government could help with things like cleaning and gardening. For *free*. Isn't that *great?!* But she doesn't fall for it.

'I can clean my own house. And Dennis mows the lawns,' she says defensively.

'I know. And you both do a great job. But you've worked hard all your life, Mum. You deserve to get help.'

I explain that people could also come to assist with talking and moving more comfortably around her house. Look at areas that might be unsafe. That any help we can get for her has got to be good, *right?*

My thinking is that setting up additional help now, we can keep her at home longer as her health or cognition declines. That it's best to get in early, so she can get used to it, rather than down the track, when she may resist change because of the trajectory of her disease. I hope it never happens, but it may come to a point when caring for Mum might be too much for just Dennis and me. I like to think that if I was in the same position, I would have the wherewithal to get help, though I understand Mum's desire to maintain control. Mum has always modelled that having dignity is crucial, but that stubborn pride doesn't get you anywhere.

She looks at me evenly. 'Can they fix me?'

We both laugh. 'They can only try.'

Despite her initial resistance, it's a 'yes' to forging ahead. Once again, I'm grateful for her willingness to let people in, for her openness at giving things a shot. I suspect it's going to keep us all in good stead for any challenges that lie ahead.

GIFT #3

Humour

I will find humour in every situation

September 2020

Mum has always had a well-honed capacity to see the absurd, to find the silliness in even the grimmest of circumstances. As I try to wrap my head around government-funded aged care services, I realise I'm going to have to try very hard to channel Mum's sense of humour.

The My Aged Care website is a model of plain English simplicity, but entering and navigating the system proves to be much more convoluted. I read that applicants need an Aged Care Assessment in order to get help in their home. This determines their eligibility for a Home Care Package, which is a pool of money administered by Services Australia. The Package is redeemed as services – from meals, to cleaning, to gardening, to personal care – depending on their needs and the availability of services.

Once approved, applicants will join a queue to be allocated a Package. When this happens, they have 60 days to choose a Home Care Provider and then enter into a Home Care Agreement. While the My Aged Care website has a list of providers, it's apparent that they have different strengths, charge different rates for particular services, and have different commission levels.

Applicants may need to contribute to the cost of the program. Fees are income tested. In order to determine what the fee will be, applicants need to do an income assessment with Services Australia. A form needs to be filled out.

If applicants need help with navigating this system, they can make a face-to-face appointment with an Aged Care Specialist Officer or get in touch with OPAN, the Older Person's Advocacy Network.

Once they have a Home Care Package in place, a meeting is arranged with a Home Care Service Coordinator. This person coordinates services, answers queries and addresses complaints.

It takes me quite some time, and a few visits to related websites, to get my head around these services and how they're run. George has already been through the process of organising home care for his parents. He passes on the book *We Need to Talk About Mum & Dad* by comedian Jean Kittson. I vividly remember watching Jean perform live comedy on *The Big Gig* in the '90s, delivering whip-smart lines with her legs laced through gymnastic hoops, swinging manically across the stage. Like so many of us, she has reached the sobering age where she is parenting her parents. Though it seems there is nothing to laugh about when it comes to aged care systems, Jean has found the humour within. She gives lots of good advice and information, but the main thing that makes an impression is to *buy a notebook*. And write down *everything*, especially when you are speaking to government departments. This includes call reference numbers, form numbers and any advice you are given.

I pick up the phone and ring up a My Aged Care operator to book in an initial assessment for Mum. They tell me it's likely she won't get an appointment for a few months. And, given the restrictions, it will be over the phone. I'm asked questions about my status as her representative, about who is living with her, about whether I have power of attorney, and about setting up an online account to streamline the process. Though the operator is kind, and explains the process clearly, my head reels. I want desperately to laugh with Mum about how absurd navigating this whole system seems to be, but then I remember it's her care I'm dealing with. Not for the first time, I wonder how elderly people, particularly those with very little English, low digital literacy or those with cognitive impairments might navigate this system.

*

It's late November, and I marvel at how we survived the past few months as we careened towards the end of year.

George's Dad had a fall, breaking his elbow and a few ribs. Emmanuel completed his VCE exams. There was the usual end-of-year madness with marking and chasing up students. And I'd prepared for and presented at an online writer's conference on a

Master's thesis I'd started earlier in the year – I had barely any time to breathe, much less engage with study. The migraines I've had since primary school were coming thick and fast, but I was dosing up on painkillers and pushing through them as best I could.

Two months after we'd applied for a Home Care Package, we'd hit the top of the queue for an appointment for an assessment. The assessor was only able to talk to Dennis and me, because Mum couldn't communicate over the phone at all, even with an interpreter. The assessor said she would recommend Mum go on a Package, likely Level 1, which is low care.

Though Mum hadn't yet been accepted for a Package, she was eligible to see some allied health practitioners thanks to state-based funding. A kindly assessor had come out to Mum's home to write up a plan for Mum's care services. She said she would provide a range of referral codes for Mum to access care that was relevant to her needs, including for residential aged care. I'd told her we didn't need that code, but she gently said it would be good to keep it, *just in case*, and that it might save more work down the track.

A physiotherapist and occupational therapist had since observed Mum walking in her house and yard and down the street, getting into her bed, easing into Dennis's car. A walking frame and sturdy chair was suggested. Her bathroom was assessed for ease of access to the shower, and the lip that might be a tripping hazard was noted. A shower chair was recommended.

There are a few steps leading out into the front and back yards. Rails were measured up.

When the walker arrived, Mum had said, 'What will people say when they see me with this?' She was embarrassed. I'd reassured her that plenty of people have walkers, that it would help with making sure she is stable on her walks. But after a practice run with the physio, and a few tries with me, the walker was relegated to the lounge room.

The shower chair takes up too much room in the shower, and Mum barely fits in after it. I buy her a smaller one from the chemist. Both sit in the bath, unused.

The sturdy chair doesn't slide under Mum's table, so it gets moved to her bedroom. At least there she can sit on it to put her shoes on, but it agitates her, reminds her of a hospital or nursing home.

The rails along the steps are installed. Despite Mum's initial resistance and embarrassment, she uses them as support to get up and down the stairs. After all this work to put tangible aid in place for Mum, at least she's using *something*.

*

It's the first day of December, and a speech pathologist is sitting at Mum's kitchen table. Earlier that morning, I'd reminded Mum who was coming today: a woman who's here to help with talking; explain she is like the woman she met with after her stroke. That woman's catchphrase was *siga, siga*. Slowly, slowly. *Try and get the words out slowly. Don't rush.* We'd met with her on and off for the better part of a year. In amongst the angst of trying to find her words, there was lots of laughter. Those sessions had led to some improvement to Mum's speech and understanding, giving her enough functional language to be able to communicate her needs, hold simple conversations.

This new speech pathologist sets out her materials and starts showing Mum pictures, asking her to repeat things. She explains that these questions are to work out where Mum is at. She says that any work they do together will be about helping Mum communicate her needs as best she can, for as long as she can. In this initial session, she will write some things that are achievable in the limited number of sessions she might have with Mum – and in any subsequent sessions, she will work with Mum towards those goals.

'What would you like to get out of these sessions?'

'I want my words back … Can you do that?' She looks at the speech pathologist beseechingly, as if she can pull out a magic wand and make it all better.

The speech pathologist smiles, explains that it isn't just about words – in fact, only a small percentage of meaning is conveyed through words – it's about communicating with your eyes, and hand gestures as well. She explains that tone and body language makes up a very big part of communication. Mum is good at both those things, and the speech pathologist and I both affirm it. Mum nods, but I can see she's not convinced.

'But can you help me. With the words …'

The speech pathologist says she could get some cards that Mum could point to when she wants something. She believes that they are available in Greek, but as Mum can no longer read, they aren't that helpful.

Between us, we manage to come up with something the speech pathologist can write down in her notes: 'To be able to talk better with my family.'

*

That same afternoon, Mum has an appointment at St Vincent's Hospital in Fitzroy for an MRI. It's the final piece in the puzzle before we meet with the geriatrician to confirm if Mum has dementia. There's limited street parking, and Mum can't walk as far as she used to. We park in the multilevel car park, and as usual these days, Mum's anxiety skyrockets when she's in an unfamiliar environment. *We're going to get lost. Where is it? Do you know how to get out of here?!*

I reassure her. We come down to the ground floor and walk out past the smokers attached to drips. I've read about the hospital's long history of supporting the disadvantaged: alcoholics, homeless people, prisoners. This area was once staunchly working class, but now the nearby housing commission towers are surrounded by boutique restaurants, galleries and artfully styled giftware shops. We too have a long history with the hospital: Mum spent many months here after a serious accident; Dad in the last months of his life as they ran test after test to see why he was wasting away, why he could no longer stand. I remember the long, coloured stripes of its hallways, visiting friends and family who had been treated here over the years.

Our appointment is in an old section of the hospital, the Healy Wing. Its maze-like tunnels lead to a table strewn with antiseptic, lists and labels; red squares taped to carpet that set us in front of robotic-looking heat sensors; barcodes that send our location to a database that stores it should we be exposed to an ever-morphing virus. There are the usual questions and forms to be filled out. I'm not allowed past a certain point as Mum is led into the scan. I worry about her getting fatigued with all these diagnostic and assessment appointments. But soon after, she walks out, smiling. The nurse calls Mum a trooper, and she leads her back to the waiting room. That's another test behind us.

*

The gently spoken geriatrician leads Mum to the consulting room through a rabbit warren of hallways. It's early December and this is the last of Mum's medical appointments for the year. This is the second time we have been here, and now that all the tests have been done, the geriatrician will make the call about whether Mum has dementia. It's been eight months since we started on the path to diagnosis, with many delays due to the lockdowns. The geriatrician was a bit surprised and perturbed that my brother, as the primary carer, isn't here. When I explain that the receptionist was very firm about only one person being able to accompany Mum to appointments because of ongoing restrictions, the geriatrician can't help but betray her irritation at the ripple effect the lockdowns have had on her elderly clients.

Getting the interpreter on the laptop is a process – there are several minutes of fumbling before the interpreter's face finally appears on the screen. I'm relieved it's not someone I know. The interpreter we had at the initial appointment was known to me through my professional networks, and the personal nature of the business at hand felt awkward. During that appointment, the geriatrician had taken Mum through a series of lengthy cognitive tests. It had quickly become clear that she was unable to successfully complete many of the set tasks. The geriatrician had turned to me to find out more about Mum, about what was usual for her. Not for the first time, I talked about the challenges involved in gauging change. Mum was barely literate and had fully lost her capacity to read following the stroke. It was hard for her to follow instructions, particularly ones so unfamiliar. And all these tests were being explained to her through an interpreter via a laptop in quite formal Greek. I had felt sorry

Humour

for Mum, couldn't begin to imagine how all this testing and appointments were making her feel.

The geriatrician says there was nothing unusual about Mum's scans except for some small aneurisms and other minor abnormalities that were not unusual in someone of Mum's age. However, the changes in functionality – her continuing loss of language, having lapses where she momentarily forgets where she is, an inability to perform most of the tests, sleep disturbance and difficulty with complex tasks – indicate that she has dementia. And that it is likely vascular in nature. This means that it is caused by restricted blood flow to the brain. She tries to explain things as clearly and succinctly to Mum as possible, her tone firm but reassuring. 'You have dementia, Chrisoula. This is not a reason to feel bad. The changes are likely to be very slow. There is no medication that can cure this. There is a medication that may help you with word finding. But I believe it is not wise to use this in your case, as it may give you mild seizures. And there is no guarantee that this medication will help.'

She pauses between each of the statements, gives the interpreter a chance to catch up. Mum nods, seems to understand. Her demeanour appears resigned: this is yet another thing to be endured.

The geriatrician turns to me. 'What is more likely to help your mum now is making sure she has good support, and that she maintains her overall general health such as managing cholesterol and blood pressure to reduce the risk of strokes.'

The geriatrician notes Mum's weight, which is still in the healthy range despite a slow decline over the years, and makes another appointment in a few months' time. She says she will send a letter formalising the diagnosis.

We walk out into the sunshine. It feels as if something should look different now that the diagnosis has been confirmed, but the street looks the same. I feel strangely calm, have become adept at putting my emotions to one side so that I can process information, be helpful for Mum.

I take Mum's arm, and we slowly make our way to the car and back home. The geriatrician's words echo in my mind. *You have dementia, Chrisoula. This is not a reason to feel bad. The changes are likely to be very slow.* The take-home message? Nothing is going to happen in a hurry.

*

It's early April 2021, and I've taken myself off to the seaside town of Mt Eliza to lick my wounds.

There wasn't much respite at the start of the year. The letter had arrived confirming Mum's diagnosis, and it got filed away along with the many other bits of paper documenting Mum's care: a large folder had grown into two. I'd worked on a Master's thesis during the holidays, all the while feeling resentful that I couldn't have a proper break to catch my breath. There were visits to Mum's and my in-laws, Christmas to be celebrated, Mum's birthday and Emmanuel's too, and then a commemoration of 16 years since Dad's death. There had been a flurry of meetings to prepare for the start of the teaching year. Mum's arthritic knee required an x-ray, and we had to see to her sore tooth and loose dentures. In between, I'd managed the odd visit to the beach with George and the kids, which felt like a luxury after so much containment in our local surrounds. But the joy was short-lived: in February, there was another short lockdown, and we were to continue to work from home for the foreseeable future.

I've recently dropped out of the Master's in order to prioritise Mum's and my family's care, and to maintain my sanity. I am both relieved and disappointed. This Mt Eliza retreat is a desperate bid to say good riddance to 12 horrible months. I'm feeling the need to step outside of myself and my daily life to see things a little more clearly, to give myself space to honour my need, my compulsion, to write. I've spent the past year feeling creatively constipated, as if too many words are stuck inside me.

But instead of writing, I'm walking the beach at sunset, feeling a little lonely. There are parents with their young children, small groups, and I can't help feeling sad that our children aren't that little anymore. Two small girls tell me their names, report that their brother needs a haircut. Their harassed mother just smiles wryly. I don't miss the tiredness, the constant-ness of my children being this young. But still, my long-yearned for time away from home, time to dedicate to words, now feels a bit empty. Why can't I just be content?

When I finally settle into a routine, I find myself writing about Mum. About the ritual of putting on pants that aren't bound by elastic, about applying a peel of red lipstick, and visiting her once a week to cook her lunch – in the end, it becomes a love letter of sorts. As the words multiply and slip from me, and tears leak at surprising moments, there is a sense of coming back to myself. I creep around the edges of the malaise I've been feeling this past year. I edge around it quietly, stealthily, so as not to scare it away. I want to get to know it, to befriend it. It is part of me, and I need to embrace it so that it doesn't hit me over the head when I'm not looking.

*

I ring Mum as I walk around the Mount Eliza foreshore. I don't tell her I'm not home with my family, as she will worry. *What am I doing on my own at the beach, without my family?*

Mum talks about our recent gathering at Easter, where my in-laws, sister-in-law, her partner, her wheelchair-bound mother, and our immediate family had lunch at ours.

After Mum compliments the food, how nice the house is looking, and the company, she laments that she didn't bring anything, couldn't be more helpful. '*Einai ligo skoteino,*' she says. It's a little dark.

Mum often reminisces about when she met my father-in-law, Alfred, nearly 20 years ago now; how tall, how strong and very

Humour

straight he was. And my-mother-in law, Doris – now there was a real *kyria*, a lady. There were visits to each other's homes, beers cracked open, meals shared. Now my in-laws are both bent over, unable to walk without aids. Toileting, eating, even talking, is a challenge for my father-in-law. My mother-in-law looks at him concerned, shakes her head; it's too much trouble to come out. 'Never again,' she says each time we organise a gathering.

Arranging a visit for my in-laws to our home is an exercise in tightly orchestrated logistics. My father-in-law needs to be dressed for the weather, his medications given in a blister pack, his wheelchair, toileting seat and continence aids packed. George picks his father and his accoutrements up from the care home, then swings by his parents' home to pick up his mum – with her walker joining the equipment in the boot. His sister's partner, Monica, needs to organise a wheelchair taxi for her mother well in advance. The return trip by taxi is timed so that her Mum doesn't have to go to the toilet. This requires another specialised chair that isn't portable. Mum, who is the most mobile of all, needs constant reassurance for days leading up to each social event. *It doesn't matter that you can't say all the words. Just do the best you can. Most people understand you perfectly well. Don't worry. Don't worry. Don't worry. It's Happy Easter, not Merry Christmas. Happy Easter. But don't worry about it. No one really cares.* On repeat.

When George pulls up, we help my in-laws out of the car, get their equipment out and start the balancing act that is getting them up the single step into the house. Inside, there's a confusion of chairs and walkers and *Happy Christmases* and *Merry Easters* as Mum and Dennis and the kids greet my in-laws. We seat everyone. We have made a special effort with the table – yellow daisies grace the middle; individually wrapped cups of Easter eggs nestle in a bed of yellow fluff, Easter-themed napkins finish off the look. Since any one of these celebrations could be the last, small rituals and details feel all the more important. Josephine, George's sister, brings traditional Maltese sweets. The bench is laden with food. We toast to good health, to continued gatherings. But we all know that the gatherings are finite. Who knows how many people will be here at the next one?

On returning to Melbourne, I visit Mum, watch for signs that the darkness she spoke about last week isn't hanging over her. But she is just glad to see me, and soon we are cooking and giggling. Even though it is a little dark at this time, I'm relieved that she can still find something to laugh about.

GIFT #4

Warmth

*I will have a warm hug ready
when you need it*

October 2021

Though the lockdowns have continued on and off, the bulk of the year passes without too many dramas. I continue to visit Mum every Friday, schedule extra time for vaccinations and medical appointments. After the chaotic activity involved in diagnosing her condition and setting up supports, it feels as if things are finally settling. I recall the geriatrician's words: *The changes are likely to be very slow.* I'm relieved that Mum's behaviour appears largely stable.

But the respite for George and I when it comes to caring for our elderly parents doesn't last long. There's been a coronavirus outbreak at the aged care home where my father-in-law lives. Two days after the first case is discovered, there are 12 confirmed cases, with numbers rising daily. They've been so careful with policing visits and contacts with the vulnerable residents within. They dodged the deadly outbreaks last year. But despite their best efforts, the virus has entered the barracks. And now it's war.

The residents need to stay in their rooms. Each day they do a RAT, every second day a nose and throat swab. Staff are back in full protective gear, where I imagine them sweating it out as they zigzag from room to room, showering, feeding, taking the temperatures of the residents within. My father-in-law tests negative over a few days. The longer he's in, the higher the chance of him catching the virus, of his mental health declining once again.

The wheels start turning to get him back home until this blows over. There, he will need 24-hour care. A schedule is drawn up. George and his sister Josephine will tag team to stay with their parents. Food deliveries, sanitary products, a wheelchair and shower chair are the bare essentials they need – the rest can wait. The wheels are set in motion with admirable speed.

On Monday morning, my father-in-law is packed and ready to leave. The nurse assures us that he should be okay to go, though his latest swab results haven't come in. George shoots out the door to pick him up.

An hour later he calls.

'Is everything okay?' I ask.

'Well, no, not really. Dad came out. He didn't look at all well. Sounded kind of chesty. We sat in the car, did a RAT test. And it came back positive. He has to go back in, and I have to isolate …'

I start laughing. I know this isn't the most appropriate response. But I can't help it. The last 17 months have been spent avoiding this very situation. Masking, sanitising, distancing. Discussing case numbers, infection and vaccination rates over the dinner table. Missing out on meeting newborns, attending funerals and celebrating milestone birthdays and anniversaries – all in the name of keeping this disease at bay. It's a reminder that despite our best efforts, we have so little control. I can't help but think about Mum – how will this impact her? I don't want Mum's care to fall down the priority list. But I can't worry about that now – I need to address the problem at hand.

Even as we nut out a plan, laughter slips out of me in slightly hysterical blips and gasps. My husband will drive to a Covid testing station. Our toilet-less, kitchen-less garden studio is to become his quarantine home for the next two weeks as per government regulations as he is considered a primary contact. I will get the camping mattress down, move out my work equipment so that he can isolate. I laugh. It's absurd. The whole goddamn situation, this one we have been doing our utmost to avoid, is absurd.

For the next hour, I go back and forth between the house and studio with toilet paper, kettle, toiletries, towels. I pull down an antique potty and baby bath transported from Malta that haven't seen the light of day since our children were toddlers. Biscuits. A book. I bark out grumpy instructions to Dolores and Emmanuel. They comply, argue about how sensible this plan is. Maybe Dad should isolate in a hotel? I argue that it's only temporary pending results. *We will see. Let's take it day by day.* They are not convinced. Dolores retreats into her online classroom, brows knitted.

Warmth

By the time George gets home, the studio is ready for him to feasibly spend the next two weeks. The kids and I look out the kitchen window, watch him come into the backyard. I've stopped laughing. Instead, I make my daily call to Mum, take solace in hearing about her gentle routines, bask in the warmth of her voice. At her house, nothing has changed. I don't tell her about George, or his dad. What good would it do for her to know?

*

The next morning, I see a light on in the studio. I take a tray of breakfast out, and leave it on the table between the house and the studio, a contagion-free no-man's land of sorts. There have been no phone calls in the night, no changes to report. I see my son off to work, then George and I chat on Messenger, do the crossword. He hasn't got any symptoms. I get load after load of washing out, empty bins and do dishes, teach a class from my laptop. In the online classroom, it's like I'm talking to myself. My jaunty tone, one that's designed to lift the mood, feels foolish. I quip that I have to laugh at my own jokes. I have no idea if my students respond to my self-reflexive humour – their cameras and microphones are off.

Later that afternoon, my father-in-law's doctor calls. He is ringing from his home, where he too is isolating after being a close contact of someone with Covid. He reports that my father-in-law has a temperature. That he is being managed with steroids and vitamins. Though he feels unwell, he is still managing to ask for chocolate and milk. This is a good sign.

The aged care home provides daily progress reports. George is reassured they have plenty of oxygen available should it be needed. He's told that the carers are sleeping on site, worried about spreading infection if they leave the premises. Doctors in full protective equipment are visiting from a nearby hospital. However, should residents get very sick, they will not be moved to hospital. Nearby hospital beds are full and there are not enough ventilators.

I visualise my father-in-law, lying in his bed, not fully understanding the need to isolate. George and I agree he is around people who are familiar to him. People who will care for him as well as they can. But not the people who love him.

When we talk about it, over the phone, both our voices break.

'I'm sorry,' he says.

'Why are you sorry? I'm sorry for you, and for Papa. You can't be with him … I just want to give you a hug,' I say to George.

'Me too,' he says.

Though hugs don't solve anything, they always seem to help. There's something about the reassurance of touch, of feeling safe in someone's arms. I recall Mum's embrace when I was a child, her warmth and smell as I snuck onto her lap, wrapping my arms around her ample waist. Now we have come full circle – I have to stoop slightly to fold Mum in my own arms. In doing so, I convey my love for her as she did to me all those years ago.

I come back to the present. It's only day two of isolation. Any hugs between George and I will have to wait.

*

A few days later, I visit Mum with a tray of food in hand. I still don't tell her about George quarantining or about my father-in-law being unwell. I don't want to worry her unnecessarily. She's been to the chemist to pick up her medications, and they've taken her blood pressure, which is high. Though she doesn't want to go, I make an appointment with her doctor for later in the afternoon – I'm hypervigilant about blood pressure, which is a risk factor for strokes. Thankfully, by the time we meet with her doctor, all is back to normal. Mum is okay. I can go back to stoking the home fires.

Some days later, George gets a phone call from the Department of Health. They read out a lengthy script outlining his obligation to isolate as he was exposed to someone who was Covid-positive. They don't ask him for the results of tests or his vaccination status or how he is. Later that afternoon, two stern-looking women in blue uniforms come to the door with a tablet in hand, here to check whether George is isolating. George comes out from the studio. When he walks towards the porch, masked, they both take a few steps back. They confirm his details, leave a few minutes later. He complains that they didn't ask him about his wellbeing. We laugh. As long as he's isolating, his wellbeing is of little importance.

A few days later, George video calls me. The hospital doctor, who is looking after his dad and other residents, called. His father's oxygen levels have gone down from 80% to 70%, his sugar levels up. He is pulling out the air tubes they have inserted. Likely they will need to take him to hospital to put him on a ventilator. George looks up at me, back at his notes. He can't believe it. His father was on the mend. He'd not been on oxygen tubes yesterday.

'If his oxygen levels keep going down at this rate, he could die …' The sentence hangs in the air. George looks back at his notes.

'George. Are you okay?'

'Yeah, look, I'd better get off the phone. The doctor said he would call back.'

Ten minutes later, George calls again.

'They got the wrong patient. Dad's fine. His oxygen levels are at 95%. The only thing wrong with Dad is a few mouth ulcers, and his mental health …'

'That's great. And terrible. How could they get it so wrong?'

George shakes his head as if to say, *It's war out there.*

*

On our morning calls, George talks about when all this blows over, he and his sister might need to think about moving his father to a Covid-free aged care home. I say I can't deal with conversations about plans for next week, or the week after. I need to think about today. About going for yet another Covid test, so I can see my mother-in-law tomorrow in lieu of George visiting. So that I can visit my own mother, who is at risk of falling to the bottom of too many pressing priorities. My marking is banking up like a slow-burn headache and I can't seem to get any traction. I'm trekking across the garden several times a day, delivering food, towels and drinks, taking back washing that needs to be sterilised. I can't even manage a half-hour walk around the block to clear my head. The phone notifications beep constantly – George needs this, he needs that. After a while, I switch these off – it's more than I can deal with.

When I visit my mother-in-law, she is distressed about George. I tell her he is still working, is listening to music and watching movies on the computer at night. He has even cleaned the garage. To me he seems more relaxed than he's been for a long time. It's clear that taking a break from caring is doing him the world of good.

It's true that George was having a great time the first week, but this soon wears off in the second week. George laments that it's been too long since he's visited his mother. His sister is exhausted from holding the fort, and him being dependent on me and the kids for everything is losing its novelty. The times between his requests and our responses to them are getting longer and longer. Several days in I implore him to come in, argue that it's very unlikely that he has Covid. But he insists on seeing it through.

On day thirteen of George's isolation, the Department of Health calls again – the rules have changed. Now, only one week of isolation is required. It's strange when he walks across the garden. We are awkward with each other. We don't kiss or hug after many days of being so diligent with infection control.

That night, we get a call from the aged care home. My father-in-law's oxygen levels have dropped. They need to take him to hospital. George sits at the kitchen table, has a long three-way discussion with his sister and a paramedic. They won't take his dad to hospital until everyone is clear about my father-in-law's end-of-life plan, drawn up some months ago. The paramedic wants to confirm that everyone understands the implications of what is written therein: there will be no resuscitation should my father-in-law lapse into unconsciousness. The paramedic sounds unsure of himself, fumbles with the wording, as if he is reading from a script that's shaking in his hands. George writes everything down in a notebook. It feels as if his dad's life is in his and Josephine's hands.

'Is my father dying?' George's voice reverberates loudly in the quiet room.

The question leads to more prevarication by the paramedic: *he can't say, it's not something he can comment on …* I sense

Warmth

George's fear and frustration: he can't just hop in the car and meet the ambulance at the nursing home, see for himself what is going on. When he gets off the phone, I give him the only consolation I can offer: a listening ear and a hug.

An hour later, we get a call from the hospital. They too confirm that should my father-in-law's condition worsen, there will be no ventilator or CPR administered, as per his stated wishes. The operator there is much clearer, has a firm and reassuring voice. 'No, your father isn't dying. We just need to make sure everyone understands the repercussions should his condition get worse.'

It's a wakeful night. The next day, George's dad seems to have improved somewhat. We are reliant on hospital calls for updates, as they rarely pick up when George calls. A few days later, his dad is transferred back to the care home.

More than a dozen people in the home have died over the past few weeks, but he's pulled through yet again. The 15-minute visits from the window can recommence. George is back to visiting and caring for his mum, and I can turn my attention more fully back to my own mother. It feels as if we've weathered another big storm. But we're all mentally exhausted. The laughter of a few weeks ago feels like a long-distant memory.

*

With the dramatic events of George's dad behind us, we are back into some semblance of routine. After the recent clean up at Mum's house, I'd found some pants in her bungalow that fit her, but they need hemming as they are too long. I get her to try them on, lean down on the floor with pins in my mouth, just as she has done for me on so many occasions. I adjust them to the right length.

She insists on hemming them herself. I watch her try, unsuccessfully, to stitch the hem loosely into place in preparation for machining. After several attempts, and mounting frustration, I ask gently if she would like me to try. She nods. Donning my reading glasses to thread the needle, I start to hand sew, stitch by stitch. She watches me, proud but sad.

'What has happened to me? I can't do anything anymore!'

'Oh, Mamma …' There is nothing I can say that will make this better. I don't want to give her false reassurances. I give her a hug instead. She leans into me, small and vulnerable.

I say I know someone with a machine who can sew them for us. It's not exactly a lie – I just don't tell her that I will have to pay for them to be sewn. She agrees that would be a good thing, and I put the pants into a bag, try to shift the focus as I once did with my young children when I wanted to distract them: *Perhaps it's time for a drink?* We make our way to the kitchen.

Afterwards, I drop the pants off to a local repair shop. It feels wrong, on principle, to hand over a sum that would cover the cost of a decent second-hand machine.

And so I find myself visiting a stranger's home as the light settles into a grey dusk. A woman answers the door, calls out to a man working at the kitchen table. He puts his laptop down, skirts around their young son, and comes out to show me to the garage.

He doesn't have just one sewing machine to sell, but several. He's selling them on his mum's behalf. She started buying them and couldn't stop, he tells me. After spending all morning looking at sewing machines online, I can understand the addiction. I'd salivated at antique Singers, Vickers and Rushbys. The lockdowns, and the need to source a sewing machine to keep sewing now that Mum can't, has brought me to this suburban garage. I may get a hefty fine for breaking lockdown rules, but I'm determined to come away with an operational sewing machine.

Now, looking at machines on the floor of this man's garage as the light fades to dusk, a tsunami of memories washes over me.

I am nine years old. Our family runs a fish and chip shop in Heidelberg. We live in the back of the shop. Mum's sewing machine is in the front room, and I'm sitting on the chair, eager to work it. Mum is leaning over me. She is showing me how to insert a piece of fabric under the presser foot, warning me to avoid the sharp needle, her hands over mine to help turn the handwheel. It resists against my small hands, requires effort. I beg her to let me turn the machine on, but she refuses – it's too fast, I'm too little. In this painstaking way, I slowly sew small pillows for my dollies, or simple purses to place the coins I occasionally nick from the cash register. My efforts are awkward, lopsided, but Mum comes in and out between the lunch and dinner time rushes, compliments me, encourages me to keep going. No doubt it is a way of keeping me from under her feet, but I can tell she is proud that I am interested in her craft.

As a seamstress, Mum appreciated well-fitting clothes, recognised quality fabrics from afar, and always encouraged me to dress to flatter my body shape no matter the fashion. We shared the same pear-shaped bodies, much to my chagrin as I grew into a teenager. But she was nonplussed. *This is what we have been given. It's up to us to make it look good.*

I'm transported to another time, several years later. We have moved back to our home in Collingwood, the fish and chip shop sold. I am 13 years old. There's a Greek dinner dance at the Collingwood Town Hall. Mum has made my cousin Kathy and me halterneck summer dresses in a large polka-dot print. We walk up and down the foyer of the stately old hall, making any excuse to go to the toilet, get some air, take a break from the heaving dance floor. At the cusp of childhood and womanhood, I feel so *sexy*. I'm sure my cousin feels it too. We glance furtively at boys in dark pants, white shirts and thin ties. We admire our own reflection in the gilded mirrors in the bathrooms. Our pointy stilettos pinch at our feet, and we take it in turns to wear Mum's faux fur because it's too cold for summer dresses. How naïve, how hopeful we were.

As Mum sewed, she would often tell stories of studying to be a seamstress in Greece, of going to the neighbouring town of Kalamata for her apprenticeship. Later, she had her own apprentices crammed into the front room of her stone village home. By all accounts, she was successful. But her sewing machine was given to her older sister as part of a dowry. And with two younger sisters of marriageable age without dowries, Mum undertook to migrate to Australia to ensure all their futures. It wasn't the first time, nor would it be the last, that she would sacrifice her own needs for the good of her family.

In Australia, things changed. Her passport still read 'seamstress', but the work here was very different: she sewed towering mountains of nighties in factories, and then, afterwards, in her bungalow in her backyard. Though she wasn't paid nearly as much, and had to put in 14-hour days, she preferred to work from home, to continue to care for us, make meals, clean up after us all. She often had sore shoulders, arms and lower back, but she rarely complained.

I remember her and Dad's pride at being able to afford to purchase a second-hand industrial overlocker, rather than using the factory-supplied one.

'One day this will be yours, Spiridoula.'

That very machine stands in Mum's bungalow, and leaks oil onto the concrete floor. My brother and I decided not to fix it. It is now too fast, too powerful for Mum to negotiate.

As I look at the machines in this suburban garage – a tan-and-cream model with an '80s vibe, some ubiquitous newer models – I wonder where the woman who owned them is now, whether she is in a care home or has died. It feels rude to ask. I suspect this man just wants to get back to his laptop and his family, so I fight back my curiosity and hold my tongue.

I return to the Singer machine that first caught my attention. It's still got some tangled threads in the side compartment, a spare bobbin and some pins, as if someone just left it mid-job. The man plugs it in. When I see that it works, I pay for it and lug it to the car. Though I could have bought a brand-new machine, I'm pleased with this one, with its weight and history. I imagine using it, and Mum watching over me, approving, guiding, as she did when I was a little girl. What she has taught me, the hours I spent by her side, will no doubt kick in. I will hear her voice, encouraging me as I take up a hem, make a simple garment for my own daughter. On the floor of that garage, I could almost *feel* her handing over the baton. *It's your turn now. You can do it, Spiridoula. Keep going.*

*

Mum and I visit Dad's grave, which nature has taken over: the matches we use to light the candle and incense are soggy, cobwebs criss-cross the corners of the headstone, and its marble surface is covered in dust. The fake flowers that usually live in vases on the grave are strewn several metres away or have disappeared altogether. I place a fresh posy from our garden, wonder how long it will last in this wind.

Warmth

Because of the continued sporadic lockdowns and Mum's declining health, it's been some time since we've visited the site together. As it's walking distance from our home, I've been coming on my walks around our suburb, but I too haven't been in recent weeks.

I'd meant to come a few days earlier to clean the grave so that Mum didn't have to see it this way. I'm the custodian of the keys that open the small cavities at the foot and the head of the grave: today I've left these at home. I lament my tardiness and lack of foresight.

I wipe down the grave and its grimy cavity as best I can, vow to come back soon to give it a more thorough clean. Mum looks in the little box that holds the supplies, confused. She tentatively pulls out the wick she needs. She holds it up as if to say, *Where does this go?* I guide her, and she tops the glass with oil, manages to light it after a few tries. Her movements are unsure, but she perseveres. I light the incense, and its rose-imbued smoke wafts across the grave, dissipating around the surrounding plots. Soon the rituals, practised so many times, are complete.

Mum says goodbye to her husband, her voice a lament. Already, she is talking about which other graves we should visit – *Theio* Vassili, a former neighbour; *Kyria* Katerina, who was the 'nicest woman'; *Kyria* Tasia, who used to come for a smoke and chat in Mum's back bungalow.

Normally we would walk to each grave, but there are cracks in the path and waterlogged sections. To avoid Mum tripping, we drive. We brush off more cobwebs from each grave we visit. Dennis has stayed at home, happy to be divested of the need to tend to all the graves that Mum insists on visiting. There is something grounding about the ritual of lighting candles and incense, and of pushing aside cobwebs, as Mum remembers and commemorates her friends.

We get back in the car, talk about going to the still very Greek suburb of Oakleigh for a souvlaki. Afterwards, we will search for a box of artichokes. It's not quite the right season, but the chase mobilises us: we are on a mission. We have honoured the dead. Now it's time to feed the living.

GIFT #5

Love

I will work hard for the people I love

February 2022

Another year has clicked over, and Valentine's Day is spent on my hands and knees. I'm scrubbing Mum's linoleum floor, trying to give it a long-overdue thorough clean. It's one of several tasks on my to-do list. While my brush passes back and forth, I think of all the heavy-duty cleaning Mum used to do: scrubbing large rugs with a broom, using plenty of washing powder and a hose, then heaving them over the washing line on her own; taking down curtains, leaning over and bearing down with all her weight as she washed them in the bathtub; climbing onto the kitchen cupboards to scour down the accumulated frying grease on the walls and ceiling. If I can get a few jobs ticked off this weekend, I'll feel I've achieved.

In Mum's kitchen, the lino is a coffee-brown colour, curled back where its edges stop at the stove. In the passageway off it, it's cream coloured with green diamonds. In the toilet and laundry, there are several layers of mismatched lino set atop wooden floorboards. There's a gap between the s-bend and the floor, and light reflects off the concrete path outside. Water pools on the floor at the base of the toilet. Either it's leaking, or my mother has been overzealous with her ablutions this morning.

I'm scrubbing feverishly with a dishwashing brush at the brown lino. Some stains on the old floor come off, but there isn't much I can do about the curled-up edges, the yellow stains and years of scuff marks. No matter how hard I scrub at the lino, mop up the leaks, or wash down the walls, I can't bring this lovely old dame of a house, or my mother for that matter, back to her former glory.

Mum taught me that a clean house meant that you took pride in your surroundings, no matter how humble they were. My job each Saturday morning was to dust and polish the furniture. I regularly emptied and cleaned the fridge, was expected to do my bed each day and respond to requests to help out, be available for preparations for parties – as a child, these jobs made me feel useful, and I enjoyed them. As a teenager, the expectation to do them when the men in the house didn't have to, grated on me. 'We aren't in the village anymore! You work hard earning money – and you have to do the housework!' I would say to Mum. I pushed back, but nothing changed. Mum kept doing the bulk of the work, both paid and unpaid.

Now, responsible for my own home, I too try to keep a neat house, grumble at family members to keep things tidy after I've cleaned up. During times of high stress, my kitchen benches are always immaculate, surfaces clear of detritus, floors mopped, and beds done – just one small way I can maintain control.

Mum has taught me well. Though it can be counterproductive, I understand now her desire to *just get it done.*

The laying down of mismatched lino is my father's work. Even as I take in the improvised nature of his repairs, one can't help but marvel at his ingenuity. A neighbour helped lay the flooring, both men in their singlets smelling of tobacco and sweat in the heat of the summer, heaving the offcuts into the house and cutting them to fit with a Stanley knife. Our neighbour would have been paid in beers, and no doubt the talking and drinking afterwards took just as long as the laying down of the lino. At close range, it's clear that it needs more than a scrub – it needs to be replaced.

As I work my way around the floor, I pass Dad's other improvised projects – the second-hand kitchen that went in after my first overseas trip as a young adult, the cupboard doors now crooked on their hinges and the edges of laminate peeling. The stained-glass window I'd made, still intact where he had placed it in the bathroom, the ornate tiles put up by a neighbour, long dead. Where the bathroom meets the hall, the floorboards are water damaged, and the old runner is wrinkly and fraying at the edges. Still, Dad's repairs, and those of his peers, are functional. I can almost hear Dad's voice, wry and amused: *My work, it's good. It will probably last longer than an expensive renovation.* I smile. His DIY philosophy with recycled and reclaimed materials was why he was able to pay off his mortgage in a matter of years on his and Mum's labourer's salaries. My husband and I, who are both well-paid professionals, are looking to our superannuation to pay ours off. Still, everything looks tired. A home needs constant maintenance, and this one is looking neglected.

I scrub the shower down – quickly – before my mother can come in. I'm worried about her slipping, as she did a few weeks back. The shower's tiles at the base need to be replaced and sealed. Mum is somewhere in the yard, and I wonder what she is doing, if she is safe. I can see why it's hard for Dennis to get anything done.

I'm here to give Dennis a break for a few days. It's been hard for him, being Mum's full-time carer. Though he hides it well, the stress on him is clear: it can be heard in the ever-escalating bickering going on between he and Mum; in his growing anxiety when more than one simple task at a time is asked of him; and his palpable relief when I take over Mum's care so he can go for a walk or go to the shops.

Our family have sent him off to the tiny seaside hamlet of Fingal in Melbourne's Mornington Peninsula. Mum and I have planned to do some spring cleaning, shop for food at our favourite market, perhaps visit a former neighbour, who is now in her nineties. I've pitched it as an adventure, about spending quality time together. But it's a thinly veiled excuse for me to see how she's doing, perhaps to observe things that I might not pick up when visiting for the day. And to do some long-overdue work around her home. I think of all the times Mum helped me – giving me breaks to go on a date with George, delivering food so we didn't have to cook, taking the kids to kindergarten and school. She looked after our family on so many occasions, and it feels good to give something of that back, albeit in a small way.

But it's becoming clear that completing the many cleaning jobs on my list is going to be challenging. Mum has been trailing me for most of the day, trying to be helpful, like a well-meaning toddler.

Now, I find her in the bungalow, picking things up, putting them in places that make sense only to her. She has a peg in her hand, which she carries around with her like a child lugs a security blanket. When I tell her I'm going to clean the kitchen windows, she trails in after me.

I climb carefully onto the kitchen cupboards and start washing the windows down.

'I'm going to do the ones outside,' she says.

I visualise her hoisting the hose up to the windows, water pooling at her feet, her slipping. I can barely keep the irritation out of my voice.

'Just wait, Mum. I'll be down in a few minutes, and we can do it together. The window is very high …'

'It's not hard. I used to do it all the time … I'm going …'

There's a stubborn resolve in her voice.

With one hand to the window and my knee on the bench, I worry I'm going to fall over. It's probably best not to try and negotiate from this position. I imagine breaking a limb, wonder what Mum might do if that happened. She would likely panic, wouldn't know what to do. It doesn't bear thinking about.

'Mum, please …'

I watch her retreating back, swipe one final time at the half-cleaned window, and climb down. I've only been here a few hours, and already I can feel myself getting frustrated that I can't do things as quickly as I might on my own. I pull myself up, make sure that my frustration doesn't bubble over. Mum has always been patient with me, and it's not hard to reciprocate. Still, if we're going to get through the next three days, I'm going to have to let some things slide.

I trail after her. 'Mum, what about you help me get lunch ready?'

*

Dennis rings around lunchtime. It appears that the freeway to the cottage has unsettled him – it's changed since he'd last driven that way. And Fingal – well, that's in the middle of *nowhere*.

'There's no noise. And *nothing* to do!' His voice is flustered. He sounds a little unhinged.

My heart sinks. It's been a very long time since Dennis has been on a trip. While the lockdowns have now eased, they have no doubt left their mark on Dennis's mental health.

'What about that list of things to do we prepared for you? Maybe try that burger place …'

Mum hears me trying to talk Dennis down, wants to know what's wrong.

'He's just getting used to things,' I say to her.

She doesn't buy it. 'Tell him to come home.'

'He's having a little break, Mum.'

After lunch, I encourage Mum to have a lie down in the bed in the bungalow. I ring Dennis shortly after. The burger place was good. He's going to check into the accommodation. He's worried about the freeway back.

Mum gets up. She can't sleep. I tell Dennis I've got to go, but to ring if he needs to. And he should come home whenever he likes if he's not having a good time.

After having an energy drink, biscuits and fruit, I suggest to Mum we go for a walk around the block. And for her to take the walker for practice. We roll it out of her room, where it stands unused. The walk is a pleasant distraction, a circuit breaker. As we shuffle along, I think back to the walks we did just a year ago. Mum is nowhere near as alert, seems less stable on her feet. I wouldn't trust her to walk on her own now. I make a mental note to talk to Dennis about it.

Later, we go to the supermarket. It's hard to understand what Mum is looking for. She shuffles up and down the aisles, looking more and more perplexed. I play a version of 20 questions. Is it milk you want? Cereal? Great. Is this the one? It's been a while since she's bought things to send home with us, and now I know why: navigating the supermarket aisles is too hard.

*

That night, I lay out my overnight things in the room where I will sleep: Mum and Dad's former bedroom. Beside their bed is a black-and-white photo of Mum that we had scanned, blown up and framed. It's always intrigued me. I pick it up, look at it closely. In it, Mum's hair has been professionally done in a '60s bouffant. It's hard to tell if she is wearing make-up, but if she is, it's subtle. At odds with her glamourous hairdo, she is wearing a simple gold cross and what looks like a home-made jumper. Mum's gaze is away from the camera, serious and a little sad, as if already looking towards distant shores she doesn't want to go to. The photo seems professionally taken. I can't reconcile the girl from the village with this image: where might it have been taken?

It takes some time, but Mum answers my questions. The photo was taken to send to a potential beau in Canada. If his response was favourable, correspondence would start, and Mum would migrate there with a view to marrying him. When Mum learnt that the man had chosen another woman who'd sailed over recently, she asked for the photo back: she didn't want all that effort and money to stage such a photo wasted.

I can't help but think how many potential brides sent photos overseas, and how things might have turned out differently for

Mum. Her fate, and that of so many women like her, depended on the whim of a potential beau, and on the countries to which the various ships needing cheap labour sailed: Canada, the US, Australia.

'Did you mind that you came to Australia in the end?' I ask.

'It wasn't my first choice. It was too far away. When I arrived, everything was so different. I cried for months. I missed my family, my home. But as with anything, you get used to it ...' She shrugs, as if to say, *What can you do?*

I am familiar with her story: bringing her two sisters out from Greece, marrying Dad, seeing her sisters wed, having children ... all the while, dreaming of returning home one day. But there was no other choice but to adapt. I think back to her first and only trip back to Greece, where saying goodbye to her family was so re-traumatising, she vowed never to return again. And she never did.

As a young woman, newly out of university, I had a strong compulsion to travel to Greece. I stayed with people who loved and knew my parents. People who told me stories about them, who showed me the rooms they ate in and the beds in which they slept. The yards they gossiped in and the fields where they collected olives and grapes and tomatoes. The sea in which they swam and the taps from which they collected water. The tables at which they ate. I saw where Mum scrabbled to finish her siblings' leftovers: she was always hungry. These items and places brought me closer to my parents, helped me understand them.

I marvel yet again at the tenacity of Mum as a young woman. She, who had never travelled further than the next biggest town, had managed to travel to, and build a life, on the other side of the world. Marry, raise children, work hard in a menial job, lose her parents and a sister in Greece, help raise her grandchildren, lose her husband, and then deal with her own ill health. All that, *and* she managed to get her photo back.

*

Later that night, helping Mum prepare for bed takes some time. I see that it's a struggle for her to undress. She is agitated, confused.

'Help, help, I can't get this dress over my head.'

Once the dress is off, I get her a glass of water, put a denture cleaning tablet in. She removes her teeth, looks at the glass, perplexed. She looks at me, and I nod. She drops them in. We both smile, but my heart aches for her.

'How do I turn this light off?' She turns to the lamp, tries to find the switch. 'Oh, how did this happen to me? I forget things …'

On kissing her goodnight, she says, 'Look after your brain. And those angels of yours … I don't know if I will wake up in the morning.'

By the time I put my weary limbs into the bed, I want to burst into tears – but they don't come. What will I wake up to in the morning?

Twelve Golden Gifts

*

In the middle of the night, Mum pokes her head into my room, ostensibly to see if I'm okay – and is happy to be gently led back to her room.

Getting dressed in the morning is challenging, but she is less tired and seems to manage it once I've laid down some clothes. I make her breakfast – toast, an egg and cornflakes – and she finishes it all, which is pleasing. Her appetite is still good. The plan is to visit *Theia* Georgia, our former neighbour in the inner-city suburb of Collingwood. It will be good to get out.

Often when visiting *Theia*, we will swing by my childhood home, which is a few blocks away. The doorbell is still the same one my parents installed in the '80s. The height of fashion then, it now evokes grubby retro chic. The house façade hasn't changed much either, but a second storey appears to have gone up where our handkerchief-sized yard used to be. The path that runs along the side of the house – where we learnt to ride our bikes; made makeshift 'slip 'n' slides' with garbage bags, a hose and dishwashing liquid when our cousins visited in the hot summer months – is now closed off with a gate.

The house was so open then: its boundaries porous, windows and doors always ajar, a passing parade of visitors and neighbours endlessly popping in for coffee, sweets, gossip. There was so little space, yet somehow Mum and Dad accommodated everyone – across from Mum's sewing machine in the tiny tin bungalow, in the concrete yard on a hot day, around the laminate table and vinyl chairs in the kitchen. She could make a family meal stretch to accommodate those dropping in. Mum had a way of making everyone comfortable and welcome, a way of making them talk – a strategic question here, a pause there – and her guests were off, telling her stories, making revelations, sharing secrets.

There was the small kitchen, where, on one memorable occasion, my cousin Kathy and I cooked sugar syrup to make toffee cups. Kathy's sister Dim impetuously dipped her fingers into the pot for a taste, screaming down the hallway and out onto the street in pain. On another day, Kathy and I sat in the backyard, finishing off a whole box of overripe passionfruit brought back from the market. Our mothers seemed always to be giggling in the background, or taking off up the street to shop, while we were happily left to our own devices: concocting simple recipes, going to the park, taking it in turns to ride Dennis's and my bikes. Our mothers often had furtive conversations about recalcitrant husbands, who they always seemed to be trying to avoid. They just wanted to be together.

When we get to *Theia* Georgia's, I swing open a rusty gate onto a tiny front yard. Though there's an old table and chairs covered in grime and detritus, the geraniums and roses in tins and pots are freshly watered, their soil dark and weed free. No one uses the front door: if *Theia* is home, the side gate and back doors are always open. The thin strip of garden that follows the path along the house is packed with herbs, a lemon tree, and newly laid tomato seedlings covered under glass to protect them from the morning frost.

We make our way to the backyard, calling out loudly to announce our arrival, which we have done countless times before. Not for the first time, I worry about possible intruders to the house. Often, we have walked all the way into *Theia*'s kitchen and loungeroom before she knows we are even there. The boundaries of this home, too, are permeable: neighbours drop in every day; her nephew stays in regular contact and helps manage any medical emergencies; and paid helpers ensure she is rarely alone for any length of time. As far as I know, she has never been robbed.

She comes out to greet us, puts an arm through Mum's, and leads her inside the kitchen. There, it's pleasantly chaotic: a bowl on the kitchen table overflows with paperwork and medicines; the kitchen benches are a carnival of bowls filled with fruit and vegetables; and a *kandili,* a votive candle in oil, surrounded by commemorative cards from the many funerals she has attended over the years.

Theia is quick to share stories from the past: of my hopping on a stool to make Greek coffee before I could properly pronounce the word *kafe*; of her taking Dennis and me on a tram to go into the city for the day; and of my ringing her as a young child, pretending Mum was sick so that she would hurry over – Mum would have a plate full of *tyganopitara* (fried bread) and feta cheese waiting for her. Mum wasn't sick at all. She just hankered for company.

Men played cards well into the night to celebrate *Theia*'s husband's name day each New Year's Eve, and a motley crew of kids of all ages hung around the lounge and the front gate, bored. It's hard to believe that was more than 40 years ago. Now her husband is buried some 50 metres from my own father, and Mum and I often light the candle at his grave.

Theia brings out biscuits, and I offer to make Greek coffee. She talks loudly, and Mum listens and nods, adds the odd snippet. Mum can't speak clearly, and *Theia* can barely hear – it works perfectly.

Theia promises to give us one of her renowned *spanakopites*, spinach and cheese pies, before we leave. These she makes with home-made filo pastry that's been rolled out on the table in her backyard. One year, she and a neighbour of hers showed me how to make them. George photographed her, and I wrote her story for a magazine. Another time, she shared the stage with me at a Greek street festival. Mum had also shared the stage, made her *tyganites patates*, fried potatoes, Greek style. I marvel at their willingness to help, to give of themselves. When I remind her of these events, and how she owned the stage, she laughs.

'Anything for you, Spiridoula,' she says.

I sit back and let the conversation, and the unconditional, familiar generosity of *Theia* Georgia's house, wash over me. It's like coming home.

*

It seems that the only time I see family friends from my father's side are at funerals. The parents of family friends and relatives are all getting sick, dying one by one. Where once we convened at weddings and baptisms, now we meet at funerals.

Today, Mum and I are at the funeral of Tina's mum Efrosini. Tina and I would spend many hours talking about our mothers during our long walks around a local lake – hers was diagnosed with dementia a few years before mine. When it became apparent that it was no longer safe for her widowed mum to live alone, she had moved in with Tina and her family. When her mum's wandering left them searching the streets on a couple of occasions, they decided the time was right to admit her into an aged care home. We'd only recently talked about her mum's steady decline over the past few months: her mum had gone from walker to wheelchair, from eating independently to needing help to eat. In the last few weeks, she had refused food, and, finally, water.

At the funeral wake, we sit at a big round table with family friends. I pile Mum's plate with food as it comes out of the kitchen. While the hall is loud and busy, she seems to be coping. She is sitting next to an aunt who is nearing 90. This aunt has heart problems and is caring for her husband who just came out of hospital following a car accident. He too uses a walking stick, and his face has a yellow pallor. I can't help thinking his might be the next funeral we will attend and quickly wipe the uncharitable thought from my mind. Any of us could go at any time. The man's son, who sits on the same table, has just had heart surgery.

I sit next to my cousin Konstantina. Our fathers were close friends in their village, and we've always considered each other cousins, though the blood link is tenuous. Growing up, we gravitated to each other. We share a sensitive, creative nature, and a love of language and books. I've always appreciated her wry sense of humour, her way of seeing the world. She has grown a mane of curly hair that reaches to the back of her waist. It is dyed amber and looks wild, untamed. It suits her. The last time I saw her it sat just below her shoulders.

'Sorry,' is the first thing she says to me. 'Sorry I haven't called. Sorry we haven't gone on that walk we talked about … It's been a bit chaotic. The kids have moved back in and with running around for my folks …'

Her dad sits opposite us, his walking stick carefully leaning beside his seat. Her mum was too tired to come.

'There is nothing to be sorry about. Things have been a bit nuts at ours, both kids got Covid, it's been busy with looking after Mum and George's parents …'

We both laugh. Life is not settling down. If anything, our days are fuller than ever. The problem is that our bodies are ageing, but we're still trying to do the things we did a decade or two ago.

'How are *you*?' I ask.

I can't help but notice that her hands move to her chest often. While we have had several long conversations over the phone since her diagnosis of breast cancer some months ago, this is the first time I've seen her.

'Look, I'm okay. The Tamoxifen is giving me hot flushes, but apart from that, just a bit of tightness around my chest. Life has gone back to normal. It was good while I couldn't drive – I had to sit tight. But now, well, I've got to go and look for work. So yeah, that's it, cancer done and dusted!' She laughs, her hair whooshing wildly, but I know it hasn't been easy.

We talk about the rigours of teaching. The breast cancer diagnosis prompted her to leave her long-time teaching job. We talk about how the administration and preparation, the marking and politics, has a way of wearing you down in the end. And the lockdowns didn't help.

'My spirit feels tired. I hanker to do something mindless for work – maybe serving fish and chips! I'm sick of thinking,' I say.

We laugh, and she nods in agreement. Our parents worked so hard to educate us, to give us a better life, and here we are at a funeral, joking about doing the very jobs that helped them put food on the table. When the time comes to leave, we give each other a warm hug, promise not to wait for the next funeral to catch up.

On the way home, Mum and I agree it's good that we came. Mum says, as she has often done in the past, that Tina's mum was such a good woman. Mum reflects on seeing her regularly at church, at family functions, says that an unkind word never passed her lips.

I look across at my gentle mother, whose blue eyes are a little bewildered these days, but who still manages to find a kind word to say about everyone.

'You're the same, Mum. You're exactly the same!'

*

For someone who has dementia, Mum has a surprisingly good memory.

She and I are coasting along the high street of Fairfield, an inner Melbourne suburb, where decades ago we scouted for boxes of cheap fruit and vegetables, slabs of feta in brine, and whole lamb. Then, the suburb was full of new migrants with fruit trees in their front yards and vegetable patches out the back. The only places to eat out were the local fish and chip shop and a dusty Chinese restaurant.

Now there are so many options for food and drink that one wonders why you would ever eat at home at all. From kimchi to kombucha, from pad Thai to pierogi, you can travel the globe by walking the length of the street. But we never eat here because Mum doesn't believe in spending money on food you can cook yourself for a fraction of the cost. And why pay for a ready-made coffee when you can buy a whole pack for the same price?

We're here to visit Mum's hairdresser, tucked in an alley off the main drag, but first she wants to change the battery in her watch.

'I don't think there's anywhere to do that here, Mamma,' I say as we slowly drive down the street, trying to avoid jay-walking pedestrians and cars pulling out of angle parking spots. The old-school watchmakers and shoe repairers have long been nudged out by the purveyors of organic single-origin beans and the ever more exotic-sounding milks with which to mix them.

She says to turn left and then left again into a residential street. Just when we've nearly run out of road, she points to a brown brick-veneer house with a concrete yard.

'I think this is it ...' She mutters something about the man who lives here and his connection to the *horio*, village, from which a Cypriot Australian neighbour of hers hails.

'Mum, this is someone's house. They don't fix watches here.'

But she insists. Despite my embarrassment at walking up to a stranger's house, I humour her. While her brain often short-circuits these days, her instincts are still good. Up to the porch I go.

There's an electric buzzer, and a name on it which sounds more German than Cypriot. There's someone moving about inside, but they don't come to the door. After some minutes, I turn and shrug at Mum in the car. At least we tried.

A figure emerges from the side gate, leaning heavily on a walking stick, his belly straining against a stained shirt.

Love

I slowly approach him.

'Um, hello. My Mum tells me you fix watches …' I say tentatively in Greek. I start to tell him about the connection to our neighbour, but he waves the introductions away, puts out his hand.

'We fix lots of things here.'

I hand over the watch.

'Do you want us to come back later?'

'No, just stay here.' Gruff. Practical. His coffee is probably cooling on the kitchen table.

He disappears behind an old security door, which slams shut behind him. A few straggly tomato plants in olive oil drums sway in protest.

Mum looks at me from the car, vindicated and pleased. It's becoming harder and harder for her to remember the smallest things, and yet, here we are. Even at this distance, it's clear Mum's eyes are twinkling, her chins jiggling. She is laughing. Before long we are both carrying on as if we've just seen the funniest comedy act. Mum may be losing her memory, but she managed to find the watchmaker. At least she still has some control.

Several minutes later, the man returns and passes over the watch.

'It's not the battery. It will cost $25 to fix. Even then I can't guarantee it will work. Better to throw it away and get a new one for that price.'

He delivers all this advice curtly. There is no need for niceties. He has helped us by telling the truth. And his coffee is no doubt now cold.

'Do we owe you anything?'

He waves me away and closes the gate behind him.

Back in the car, Mum is disappointed that the watch can't be fixed – but she found the watchmaker, and no one can take that away from her.

*

It's July 2022, some two and a half years after the first case of Covid-19. More than 568 million cases worldwide later, I've joined the fray. My test is positive.

Though I have been unwell the past few days, I can't quite believe it. George and I agree on what is to happen next to avoid spreading infection. I take myself to our bedroom, where I'll be isolating for the next seven days as per the current government regulations.

George sees to it that I have everything I need. Masks and tissues, water and painkillers. I make sure I have my phone, laptop, diary, reading glasses and enough books to see me through.

George sends me a link with the latest government reporting and quarantine requirements. He then talks with his mum, who he visits three times a week, telling her he won't be able to see

Love

her or his father for the next seven days at least, as he's a close contact. I ring Mum, check that she doesn't have any symptoms after my visit yesterday; ask Dennis to help her with a RAT test if she feels unwell. I then ring my manager, who tells me what needs to be done to inform the students I've taught in previous days.

My throat feels like it has a razor in it, my nose is running and my head hurts. I've heard our local hospital's two Covid wards are already overcrowded, their staff exhausted and overwrought. They're directing ambulances to other hospitals, which are experiencing similar strains to their resources. I hope I don't get sicker.

Despite my fears, I can't help feeling a frisson of excitement. Seven days of doing no housework, caring or teaching. *How delicious.*

*

My symptoms are manageable. I mark assignments, finish a novel, and even get some writing done. George has been delivering meals to my door, and it's felt like a mini holiday. But as soon as I'm recovered, George is afflicted with it. I'm in a dilemma: I've committed to and paid to attend a writer's festival in Mildura, where I am facilitating a session on passion projects with two notable authors. Should I go, or cancel? It's become the running joke in our family – every time we'd commit to something joyful – a few nights away to celebrate our anniversary, the chance to mind a friend's beachside home – one of our parents would fall ill and our plans would have to be aborted. We've given up on planning anything.

George gives me his blessing to go. He says the children are old enough to look after him. We agree that I will come back early if anything changes.

The last time I attended the festival, several years ago, my colleague Jacqui and I were giddy with joy at meeting David Malouf, author of one of my favourite books, *An Imaginary Life*. This is a slim volume about a Roman poet who had been exiled, in a time and place very removed from my own. The words Malouf created, their lyrical power to move beyond the temporal realm and into the spiritual, made my heart soar when I first read it as a young woman. This writing made me realise that there were words out there that could help one rise above the banality of day-to-day existence. And here I was, standing next to him, this God of transcendence, as he spoke of writing this great work in the early hours of the morning, before marking assignments. That work had slipped out of him quickly over several weeks. As he was talking of such heady matters, I had offered him a segment of a luscious Mildura orange. He'd politely declined, and I'd retreated, abashed. When would I ever stop being like my mother, always offering people food?

Love

Now that I'm here again, I'm reminded that the landscape of Mildura – the reddish-brown hue of the earth, rusting sheds housing farming machinery, a grand old hotel, the big river that runs through the town like a lifeline – takes me squarely back to my childhood.

We spent a few years, and many summers, in the small rural town of Narrandera in New South Wales helping my uncle and aunt run their fish and chip shop. I recall the wide main street shuddering with the roar of bikies riding into town. The smell of dust and diesel and freshly shorn grass. Boxes piled high with soft drinks. My little cousin Jorge, who ran wild, and once climbed the upper reaches of the two-storey hotel next door. I recall my cousins and I swinging off the Hills Hoist, and on one memorable occasion, our mums running into an above-ground pool in their bra and girdles, nearly wetting themselves with laughter. The sisters giggling – when they were shopping, when they lay side by side on Mum's bed, gossiping, when they were on the phone to each other.

I marvel now at how Mum and Dad dislodged us from our inner-city home to come to the dusty little Riverina town. It felt like a lawless time, with most of the men there living large, gambling and drinking well into the night. I suspect Mum's motivation for going was to protect her sister, to be close to her. Mum and Dad worked incredibly long hours in the shop, and I recall hankering for Mum to come home at night. I would save all my hurts for her ears only – my little toenail falling off, complaints that we had to drink the hot milk my aunty made for us each morning, and telling her of the spats that broke out between us children. I was a sensitive child, didn't have the wild hardiness of my cousins. Mum's blue eyes reflected all my problems back to me, made them bearable: *it's not so bad, you will be okay.*

At the festival, guilt is never far away: here I am enjoying myself while George is still recovering from Covid. I haven't seen Mum since I've been ill. Still, being here is like a balm for the soul and the senses. In addition to the eclectic program of writers and performers, there are long dinners and lunches: slow-cooked pork shoulder on a crisp piece of crackling, blood oranges glistening with juice, delicate octopus tendrils dusted in flour and lightly fried.

The session I facilitate goes well – with several laughs elicited from the audience – which is good for my confidence after two years of soul-destroying online teaching. Being here feels like poking my head out into the sunshine after lying dormant through the lockdowns. I feel I'm with my tribe. There is the hint of possibility, renewal.

I've been ringing Mum daily. She seems to be pottering along. I can hear Dennis in the background, his voice agitated. He's always communicated loudly with Mum, but now they bicker even while Mum and I are on the phone. My cousin Jorge is with them, painting Mum's house, and I wonder what he makes of it all. Not for the first time, I'm worried how Dennis will cope when Mum's health declines further.

Love

It's been wonderful to step away from my life, to fill my creative cup. But after several days away, I feel like I've shirked my familial responsibilities for long enough. It's time to go home.

GIFT #6

Joy

I will take joy from small pleasures

August 2022

I never thought I would feed my mother food that was microwaved in a packet.

I've arranged a meal delivery service through Mum's Home Care Package that drops off several meals each week – lasagne, chicken casseroles, stir fries. I cook for her on days I spend at her house, drop in additional food. Our kind neighbour drops food in regularly, and Kathy drops in regularly with food Mum loves. The village has kicked in.

On my return from Mildura, my cousin Jorge had observed Mum was not eating adequately, and that she was unable even to prepare a basic meal or snack. He told me he could see that Dennis was struggling. His observations had filled me with shame and guilt – while I'd been enjoying Mildura's bountiful produce, Mum had been going without. Though I was aware they were struggling, it was clear that Dennis needed more support to manage her care.

It's been a few weeks since we've organised the food. I see that sometimes Mum doesn't like the meals. I tell her I'll look into a Greek delivery service with more familiar meals.

Joy

Dennis arcs up. 'Not another change! I'm only getting used to this one. I'm going to be like a car whose wheel falls off if you change things again!' His eyes are wild, and his voice has an almost hysterical bent.

I can't help but laugh at Dennis's dramatic outburst. The care has stepped up considerably these past few weeks: I'm here three days each week to shower Mum, help with meal and snack preparation, and to walk with Mum. We've kept up with cleaners who come once a fortnight, though Dennis prepares by cleaning up before they come. A gardener helps with the lawns. Jorge has Dennis clearing the gardens to make them easier to manage. The bungalow table is once again busy with activity: a cleaner who comes regularly joins us for afternoon tea, we eat lunch out there with Jorge, neighbours start to drop by again now that the weather is starting to improve. Mum is a bit bewildered with all the activity, but doesn't seem to be fighting it.

I can't help but admire Mum's ability to take joy from the simplest of pleasures: a meal shared around the table, with both loved ones and strangers too; her sitting on a plastic chair in her nighty and moccasins in the twilight, watching and guiding George as he plants seedlings, while the kids and I fuss around her as she has always done with us; the joy on her face when her nephew, Dim's son Nicholas, comes to change her garden taps so they are easy to turn on.

In Mum's room, we lay her clothes out on the bed together. Undies and an incontinence pad. A spencer. Pants that are easy to pull on. We sort through a few types before she finds the ones she wants. A warm jumper. She always chooses either the green or the grey one, even though she has several in different colours.

We go through each item slowly, and I resist the urge to hurry her along so we can get to the next part of the process – actually having a shower.

She looks at her bras.

'I should stop wearing these.'

'Mmm …' I reflect that it's all about comfort now, that we can afford to skip over that particular item of clothing.

At least all her clothes are in the same room now. Her jumpers were in the bedroom she used to share with Dad. She hasn't slept in this bedroom since he died 18 years ago. Her pants were in the bungalow across the yard, laid out on the industrial sewing machine.

I've folded and sorted the clothes she wears each day into neat piles, put them in one set of drawers in her bedroom so she can easily see what she wants. I've been suggesting this for months, but Mum has resisted. Finally, I'd talked her into it, and there is some logical order. It makes *me* feel a little more in control – hopefully she can find her clothes when I'm not there to help her.

She stops between each of the items, gets distracted. She starts pulling at her pants to get them off before we have laid out the clothes.

'One thing at a time, Mum. Let's get the clothes ready first so they are there when you get out of the shower.'

Joy

'What do I need now?' she says.

'What about shoes?'

She finds the same old shoes she wears most days. They're easy to pull on, but they're stained. And loose on her feet. Wearing in new shoes hurts her bunion and corns. Although we've had these problems seen to at the podiatrist, they still give her grief. I can't convince her to wear one of the new pairs that I've bought her over the years, or to get fitted for sturdy shoes that will properly fit her feet. *Don't spend money on me.* The old shoes it is.

I start to help her get her clothes off. It's strangely familiar, this easing a jumper over someone's shoulders; memories of doing it for my children when they were toddlers come rushing back. Now, my son needs to stoop down to hug me, just as I stoop down to hug my mother.

Before Mum's got her pants off, I ease her dressing gown over her shoulders. I'm careful to protect her dignity, though there is nothing I haven't seen now – her dimpled bottom, her flat breasts against her still-rounded tummy, the veins that scissor down the back of her knees, the liver spots that pepper her face and hands.

She shuffles to the shower in her oversized slippers, and I regulate the water. We've recently had the hot water service adjusted so she doesn't accidentally scald herself. She steps inside and I help wash her hair, make sure to get around her whole scalp. I close the shower door and watch her shadow through the glass. She pumps body wash onto a sponge. Washes her hair again. Pumps shampoo and washes her body. Washes her hair again. More pumping. More washing of hair. My heart sinks. Her confusion is getting worse. I don't intervene. What she is doing is not hurting her, and it's important she has some control. She eventually gets around her whole body.

Mum leans over to wash her feet, and I keep a keen eye out, ready to jump forward if I see her slipping. She straightens up, lets the water wash over her.

'*Ahh ... Ooh ...*'

'It's nice isn't it, Mum?'

It takes some effort to get her to have a shower – it's such a process these days – but once she's in, she seems to enjoy the sensory pleasure of warm water, of being clean.

I watch her turn off the water – she can still do that without scalding herself – wrap her in an oversized towel and sit her down on the shower chair so that I can dry between her toes. She giggles, ticklish. I apply cream to her arms, run my hands up and down flesh that hangs loose, the muscles worn away. I inspect her fingernails, which are permanently discoloured and dark, wonder if I need to clip them or if it can wait until next time. We have been to the doctor several times about her pink raised cuticles: she needs to wear gloves when gardening and washing dishes, but the advice goes unheeded.

I keep a running commentary going, distracting her with jokes – I think she knows what I am doing and plays along.

Joy

Back in her room, she tries to put her clothes on – she holds her pants, looks at the incontinence pad.

'What do I do with this?'

'Put the pad in the pants.'

Oh yes. She remembers now.

I watch her dress. It's slow, and she is confused at times, but she gets there.

I ask her to sit down, help her ease her shoes on. Kneeling on the floor, I need to exert myself to get the shoes over her heel. Wonder how she does this herself most days, and how long it takes her.

'*Tsk.* Oh, what has my life come to. You poor thing …'

'I'm not a poor thing, Mum. I like helping you.'

She starts laughing, watching me struggling with the other shoe. She's got me going now, and my giggling doesn't make it any easier to slip the shoe on. I don't think there are many people who might find the humour in such a situation, but my mother is one of them. I think about carers who do this day in day out, the strength they need. The patience. We have a shoehorn somewhere, but that takes too much coordination for Mum. Together, with a bit of pushing, we finally have both shoes on.

Mum's hair is plastered against her head. At least it's clean after so many washes. I sit her down in front of the mirror and start blow-drying. It's been recently cut and sits nicely despite how thin it's getting. She says yes to both mousse and hairspray.

She gets up and smiles. There's been some energy expended on both our parts, but Mum is clean, and we're ready for lunch.

*

There's a urine-soaked pad behind the toilet-roll holder. There are opened pads in her drawers. They seem unused, but I can't be sure.

Mum's sitting over the toilet, wearing three pairs of undies, one on top of the other. She takes them down and crouches over the toilet. She's not wearing an incontinence pad. She looks at me, giggles, gets me started too. I crouch over her, remove two pairs of undies, insert the pad. From this position, brown spots are visible on the wall behind the toilet.

After lunch, I encourage Mum to have a lie down, to 'give her brain a rest'. All morning she's been asking when the kids are coming – on repeat. I've told her several times that it's not until later. Not to worry. That we will get pizza. That she doesn't have to do anything. A few minutes later, she asks again.

We head to the bungalow where the old single bed is, which she uses to nap during the day. It's been there as long as anyone can remember. George would sleep in it when we were engaged, and I would sneak out to him, squishing up together, sneaking back into the house in the early morning. Neighbours would sit on the bed when visiting. Dad spent many hours in it, particularly in the last years of his life.

Joy

The walls of the bungalow are a patchwork of plaster pieces that Dad cobbled together back in the day. They're adorned with a mishmash of prints and photos: above the bed there's Dad and my father-in-law, Dad and his nephews; an image of a boot executed in charcoal done by a university friend; a lake rendered in technicolour hues from the '70s. The bungalow houses a dining table and chairs overlooking the garden, several heaters, Mum's sewing machines, a tall stack of plastic chairs, a television and side table. Every corner groans with plastic bags filled with spare things: linen, elastic, stockings and spools of thread, a sign of Mum's frugality. There is something relaxing about the room's chaotic, earthly ambience. The warmth of the sun reflecting off the greenery outside always makes me want to lie down and sleep.

Mum gets into bed, knees first, awkwardly plonking herself chest-first on the bed. She finally gets there, and I sit with her. She groans.

'Why don't I just die? What's the point?'

'Oh Mamma ...'

'Why must people die?'

'I guess if people didn't die, then there wouldn't be room for people to be born ...'

'How will it be when I die? What hole will I go through?'

'I don't know Mamma ...'

She answers her own question. 'It will be a wormhole. Just like a worm, a *skouliki*.'

Mum's image of burrowing into the earth makes sense to me in a primal kind of way: all that wriggling and pushing down into the soil, making it fertile for new growth to break through. I recall Dad's struggle as he was dying: the panting, the exhalation and intake of breath; and when his chest was finally still, the sense that he, his very essence, was gone. I think of my own efforts to bring our children into the world, the sucking in and out of air; the final push and an anxious few seconds, waiting for them to take their first breath.

Mum tries to sleep, but can't settle, asks again about the kids. I reassure her, beg her to sleep, not just so she can rest, but so that I can clean without her seeing.

I stroke her hair for several minutes until I feel her body relax, but on my way out, she says, 'I prefer to die.'

'Mamma, just get some rest.'

I go back inside to wash down the toilet walls. I scrub at the brown spots, thinking all the while about dark earth and worms, life and death.

*

I'm at my fathers-in-law Alfred's aged care home for a Christmas celebration, where a nativity play is being enacted. The characters Mary and Joseph are played by residents who are well into their eighties. They have throw rugs draped around their heads and play their roles earnestly, nodding at all the right

Joy

parts. A doll representing baby Jesus, eerily lifelike, lies askew in front of Mary's wheelchair. The archangel, made from tin, is nearly knocked over by a woman with a walker who looks like she urgently needs to get to a toilet. A chap in a midnight-blue velvet jacket walks back and forth, back and forth.

I ease my way in during a lull in proceedings. My father-in-law recognises me only when I'm almost upon him. His face lights up and he greets me loudly.

'We can talk later,' I say into his hearing aid and kneel beside his chair, trying to avoid pushing crumbs of Christmas cake and *crostoli* further into the carpet. I don't envy the poor cleaners who will have to deal with the fallout of all this festivity.

Carers keep watch at the periphery. They jump to attention when a resident threatens to fall, put a hand out to stabilise them. If someone pushes their walker too roughly, or raises their voice, they quietly take an elbow, lead them away.

One of the women who organises activities for the residents is weaving carols into the play. I wonder if she belongs to a choir as her voice soars above the chaos. It makes me think of angels. She wears a kaftan with geometric, tribal patterns, and her oversized diamanté jewellery glimmers under the functional lighting. Her kind eyes and jaunty demeanour must be a balm for many a spirit here.

My father-in-law is concentrating with rapt attention. I feel a gush of love for this man who has worked so hard in underground tunnels and on factory production lines for most of his adult life. Though his body and mind have started to let him down in recent years, he still manages to tell a mean story, is always up for a laugh. I take hold of his thin hand, give it a little squeeze. He squeezes back. His grip is still strong.

I can't help but think of Mum and how she might cope in this environment. When I visited her at home earlier this morning, she was shuffling around the house, a peg in her hand, trying to remember exactly what she was searching for. Every time I see her, another piece of her has gone. Fragments of the woman she once was have dropped away like loose plaster. I lay awake at night, worrying about making the right decision for her care. But worry doesn't change anything. I try to force myself back to the room, to concentrate on the present.

> Round yon virgin, Mother and Child
> Holy infant so tender and mild ...

The words, the heavenly voice, perhaps the sleep deprivation: before I can stop myself, I'm crying into my hospital-grade mask. I turn from my father-in-law so that he does not see. I'm here to bring him a little joy, not to upset him. Despite my best efforts to curb them, the tears continue all through 'Silent Night'.

Thankfully, no one seems to notice except the woman with the angelic voice. She sings into the microphone with one hand, brings me a chair with the other. Her kind eyes threaten to undo me even further. But then she breaks out into 'Jingle Bells', and

Joy

I manage to pull myself together. My father-in-law and I sing along loudly.

When the play is finished, my father-in-law introduces me to all his favourite people. Someone hands me a plate of sweets. We're jollied along into an improvised photo booth and photographed with Christmas headgear and a fluffy koala. We both ham it up for the cameras, make each other laugh. I smile across the room at the woman with the kind eyes and the angel's voice – I hope she knows that she has lifted the spirit of many in the room, me included.

*

I've stayed the night at Mum's, as I do more often these days, to help with bedtime and morning rituals. The night has been uneventful, and the house is quiet in the morning apart from Dennis in the shower. I'm relieved: there are no dramatic events to deal with.

I round the corner, see Mum in the laundry, staring into the adjoining toilet. I step closer. The smell of faeces permeates the small space. My heart sinks. Faeces line the toilet, are smeared on the floor. Mum is shoeless. Mum looks from her feet to the toilet, looks up at me, perplexed and ashamed.

'Don't worry, Mamma. I'll help you. Just wait there.'

I grab wipes, slide gloves on, close off the toilet, wipe Mum's feet down and gently lead her to the shower. After his initial shock at the turn of events, Dennis prepares breakfast, sits with Mum while I clean up. The morning slowly settles into a routine.

There have been several messy incontinence accidents over the past few weeks. This is another downward step. I go home later that afternoon, still reeling. Urinary accidents are one thing, but faecal another. We've had a few, and I've thankfully been here every time, can get Mum into the shower. But it's too much to ask Dennis to shower Mum, awkward and hard for them both.

The challenges that Mum faces seem to be multiplying every few days. Over the course of the summer, Mum has gone from wearing incontinence pads, which she struggled to manage, to pullups. Dennis or I now accompany Mum around the block on her walks. The doors are locked at night to stop her from going outside in the middle of the night, when she thinks it's morning. I've bought non-slip material to go under all her mats, have had a plumber adjust the stove so we can turn it off at the mains when Dennis isn't home. More and more, we loathe to leave her by herself, even briefly, as we are concerned about falls, about her leaving the home unaccompanied. She refuses to wear her personal alarm, argues she doesn't need it.

She'd recently had a small stroke after her shower. She'd come out, fumbling for the towel, her hands making repetitive grasping motions. I'd covered her, led her to her room. She was confused, unstable, balancing on furniture as she shuffled along. I'd held her hand as she talked about visiting long-gone family,

Joy

her eyes turned up at the ceiling. Was this the long feared-for moment of her dying? I'd asked Dennis to bring the phone, had called an ambulance.

Mum and I had waited for several hours in the busy emergency room, but by the time she was seen, her symptoms had passed. After a scan, it was reported that Mum had likely had a small stroke. We were told that we did the right thing by coming in, but there wasn't much that could be done, and that we could go home.

I'm now at Mum's several times a week. Dennis and I have been working well together, but the times when Mum most needs support – in the morning and evenings with waking and bedtime rituals – are proving challenging. I've been on extended leave over the summer, but I wonder how we're going to manage on my return to work.

The case manager of Mum's Home Care Package is sympathetic and helpful, but due to staff shortages, the afterhours times Mum needs the most help, and limited funding available in her Level II package, we can't get carers at those times. She explains that if we want to apply for a higher-level package, we need to demonstrate that we are using the current one to the full capacity. But how can we do that given the care workers aren't available when we need them? One of the cleaners, with whom we've formed a good rapport, and who was formerly a nurse in Japan, increases her hours to shower Mum once a week. It helps, but it's not nearly enough.

We are between a rock and a hard place. I wonder whether I should just quit my job to manage Mum's care, or at least reduce my hours. But I realise that even with my being with Mum a lot more, it feels as if this is more than Dennis and I can manage between us. And the pace of change is so fast that I wonder how things might be in a few months' time.

Over the next week, I speak to my manager about reducing my hours, but in our small team it's going to be hard to get replacement teachers at short notice. Just before the semester is due to start, a colleague has a personal emergency: his son is critically ill overseas, and he has to be with him indefinitely. Instead of reducing my hours, I step up to find replacement teachers, take on an additional class. Right now, it feels that my colleague's situation is far worse than mine.

Dennis and I start to talk more seriously about Mum going into an aged care home. Though resistant, Dennis acknowledges that it's getting very hard. I invite him to come with me to look at homes, but he says he doesn't want to. That he's okay with me coming up with a shortlist.

On the way home from Mum's, I visit my aunty, and my cousins Kathy and Jorge are with her. I talk about the mounting challenges, about our considering an aged care home. I am teary, sad. They are hungry for news, perturbed that Mum's health has come to this. I'm relieved when they agree it's a sensible plan. These are people who love Mum dearly, who want to protect her as much as I do. We all have her best interests in mind.

Joy

On the way home, I think about next steps. It's easy to know which homes to approach – there are only a handful of exclusively Greek-run homes in Melbourne. I'm determined that Mum should be around people who speak her language, understand her culture, can serve familiar food. I think this will take the sting off being in an institutionalised environment. Apart from finding the right home, now only one thing remains: how to convince Mum that the time has come to move to care?

*

Over the next ten days, I arrange visits to a few aged care homes. The first I approach from the car park, skirting its perimeter to see what 'feels' I get, but its gravelly surface doesn't tell me much. I enter the substantial reception area and meet with the client services officer. She's a confident, chatty woman who has recently migrated from Greece. She takes me around, greets the residents warmly, places a Greek newspaper in front of one. It feels friendly enough, but doors are locked behind us, and there are lopsided light fittings and a general air of unkemptness. I can't help but have flashes of *One Flew Over the Cuckoo's Nest* – a novel and movie about life in a psychiatric hospital – as we make our way around the complex.

The second home I visit feels more promising. The wife of the Greek owner is doing crafts with one of the residents. There is a pleasantly warm, homely feel in one of the common rooms.

The rooms are clean, and there's a courtyard with polished tiles. Mum always hankered to live in a house with clean, sleek lines, and I think she would like it here.

Another home I visit has untidy grounds, smells strongly of disinfectant, and I discount it quickly. The final one is nicely busy, the common room abuzz with activity. I walk along a corridor before I'm quickly whisked into the office, the financial aspects of care explained to me by the liaison officer. This particular home doesn't offer respite care. From what I've gathered, respite care can be a way for both the resident and the home to gauge if it's a good fit. Mum is eligible for 63 days of government subsidised residential respite care per year. But he assures me that if we are not happy, we can transfer Mum out, even if she is in permanent care. He says that it takes time for residents to settle; and that if they do settle and appear happy, then it's best not to move them, even if you don't think the home is ideal.

From my visits I learn that post-Covid, many Greek families are more likely to wait until their loved ones have very high care needs before admitting them in residential care. That increased government compliance – though necessary – is making it harder to run aged care homes. That though the homes I have visited mostly have Greek-speaking residents, it's very hard to get Greek-speaking staff, even from Greece.

At most of the homes, I fill out a form providing our details. There is no guarantee of a place, and one home tells me they prioritise those coming straight from hospital. I don't try very

Joy

hard to get Mum on a list at the preferred facility – I still need to talk to her for a start. And though in my head I know what needs to be done, my heart is reeling. *She doesn't want to leave her home. And I don't want her to either.*

*

Over the next week, I skirt around having the conversation with Mum about care, trying to raise it in a general way. I talk about a woman who died recently, which home she was in. Mum becomes suspicious. *How do you know about that* gerokomeio, *that care home? Have you been to visit?*

I wonder if Dennis hasn't let something slip. I sidestep the question.

'I see that maybe you are struggling, that we are all struggling. At a care home, they would give you the care you need. You've fallen a few times. I don't want you to fall, maybe break a bone …'

'I haven't fallen. When have I fallen?'

'Mum, you fell in the garden. Slipped outside the car. Under the clothesline …'

'I don't want to leave my home.'

'Maybe you could come and stay with us for a while. We could set up your own bed and room …' I've already talked about this with George. We could convert the living area into a bedroom.

'What about Dennis? Would he come too?' Her tone is challenging.

I laugh. Mum still has a bit of spunk. 'How would that go, Mum? He would stay here to look after the house!' I try to lighten the tone, but she won't be drawn in.

She looks at me straight in the eyes. 'Not yet.'

She may be confused, her dementia is getting worse, but her answer is lucid, final. The conversation is closed. *For now.*

GIFT #7

Humanity

I will help you if I can

February 2023

It's Valentine's Day, and Dennis calls. He rarely calls.

'Is everything okay, Dennis?'

'I've got something to tell you …' He pauses. 'Mum was in the bathroom. I left the room to get her pants. She fell …'

'Where is she now? Is she safe?'

'She's lying in the hallway. I can't lift her by myself …'

'Did she hit her head? Is she talking?'

Dennis can't say if she hit her head. He has covered her so that she is warm. She isn't complaining, but just can't get up. I gather that she is conscious.

'Should I call an ambulance?' he asks.

I think of the massive queues the last time I took Mum into the hospital when she had a stroke, how distressing it was for her.

'I'll be there in 15 minutes. Maybe we can get her up together. We can decide then. Just keep her talking …'

I drive a little faster than usual down the roads that connect our homes, a trip made hundreds of times. I keep Dennis on the line, ask him not to leave Mum alone. My voice is calm and firm. *This capable version of myself is getting a workout,* I think wryly.

I walk in to see Mum's legs in the hallway, her upper torso in Dennis's bedroom. Dennis must have pulled her out of the bathroom, off the cold tiles. She is nude beneath the bathrobe that he's placed over her.

We try to gently ease her up, but her body is dead weight. She starts moaning. I call an ambulance.

The operator tells me not to move her, not to give her anything to eat, that someone will be with us as soon as available, and that I can call back if anything changes. I place a folded towel under Mum's head, carefully slide an adult diaper under her. It's not the thing to do if there's a fracture, but I want to avoid causing her more pain and indignity if she wets or soils herself.

Mum lies quietly, her blue eyes looking at me beseechingly. I ask if she is warm enough, whether she needs anything. She shakes her head. I tell Dennis to pack a bag of toiletries, a nightie and slippers. He is agitated, shock written clearly on his face, but glad to have something useful to do.

The picture of what happened becomes clearer as we wait. *Mum soiled herself. Dennis gave her a shower. He dried her and left her sitting in a chair while he went to get her underwear. Told her not to move. Her feet must have slipped on the wet tiles. He should have had a mat under it. Yes, that's what he should have done …*

I reflect again how unfair it is to expect my brother to be a full-time carer. That even between us, we can no longer manage Mum's care. I kick myself, should have pushed harder to get Mum into residential care.

'It's not your fault, Dennis. This was bound to happen sooner or later …'

Time drags on. Mum wants to doze, but I keep talking to her, trying to keep her awake. When asked about pain, she shakes her head, but moans occasionally. After a half hour passes, I ring the ambulance back, ask how long they expect it to be. They reiterate that we are in the queue, that there is more demand than usual. An hour in, I ring again to tell them Mum is in pain even though she's still not complaining. I'm getting desperate.

Two young paramedics finally arrive nearly two hours after I'd made the initial call. Dennis and I step back and watch as they try to shift her out of the narrow doorway. They awkwardly ease her up to a sitting position. They are quite sure she hasn't broken her hip, as she isn't complaining of pain. They slide a device under her that blows up into a seat of sorts. It's a bid to turn her to face the shortest passage to the waiting ambulance. They ask her to bend her knees so they can swivel her around, but Mum's feet start to tremble, her face contorting. It's clear her body doesn't want to do this.

The paramedics try one thing after another to get Mum out of the hallway and onto a stretcher. We stand helplessly to one side, increasingly mortified when nothing seems to be working.

Humanity

I am not convinced there isn't a break. After more unsuccessful wrangling, the paramedics call for backup. An older paramedic comes in, quickly takes in the situation. Several minutes later, Mum is wheeled out of the house on a stretcher.

At the hospital, patients in gurneys and wheelchairs are lined up along the wall at the entrance to the emergency department. We slowly inch our way towards it, and finally Mum is wheeled into a cubicle. Efficient, overworked doctors explain what they will do to assess her. They ask questions about her history, about the fall, order blood tests and a full body scan. Mum dips in and out of sleep between tests. When she wakes, confused, I repeat in Greek over and over. *We are in the hospital. You are safe. Try to rest.*

In the night, a man is wheeled into the next cubicle. He has a bandage around his head and a brace around his neck. I make brief eye contact with a woman who appears to be his partner. Her face is pale, pinched and tired. I look away.

Mum's test results trickle in: a broken hip; a fractured rib; atrial fibrillation, which the doctor explains is an irregular heartbeat that can increase the chances of stroke; spots on the liver, which are likely blood clots. *Look and ye shall find.* At 4 in the morning, after the last of the tests, Mum finally falls into a deep sleep.

A doctor approaches the man in the neck brace. Words waft across into our cubicle: *Fractured vertebrae ... very lucky... just missed the spinal cord ... it will take time, but you will walk again.*

Several minutes later the man calls out, panicked. His foot is tingling, it feels strange. He starts to hyperventilate. The same doctor who broke the news comes to talk him down in reassuring but firm tones. I avert my eyes, count down the minutes to the hospital café opening. It's too intimate here, too much pain spilling out like blood from an open wound.

Later that morning Mum is transferred to a ward. Hip surgery is scheduled for the evening. I'm allowed to stay with her today, but after that I will have to abide by the limited visiting hours mandated by ongoing Covid restrictions – two hours in the morning and two in the evening, with only two visitors allowed per day. I worry that Mum cannot express her needs and don't want to leave her alone in this strange environment of beeping machines and bleeding humanity. *She needs an advocate.* But we can't expect the rules to be bent for us, and a nurse or doctor will ring me if they need anything.

As Mum dozes, I reflect that perhaps my fear of leaving her is more about my need to maintain control and curb my guilt. Dennis and I have cared for Mum as best we can. Helped her with shopping and dressing, showering and toileting; taken her to medical appointments and answered repetitive questions over and over. But still, we haven't been able do the most important thing of all – to keep her safe.

The day is spent beside her bed on the ward. The monotony is broken by staff coming in to try and build a picture of Mum's history. How long has she had dementia? Is she allergic to anything? Was she mobile at home? Time drags as we await surgery. At 8 that evening, we learn that it has been bumped to the next day. I feel both relieved and guilty when they won't let me stay with her – after being awake all night and by her side for 30 hours, I hanker for a shower and my own bed.

The next morning, when I arrive early, Mum appears refreshed. The nurses report that she slept well. Throughout the day, she sleeps and wakes. She is often confused. *We are in hospital. We are waiting for surgery,* is on repeat. In the early afternoon, I hold her hand as they take her down to surgery, watch the gurney disappear behind double doors.

In the early evening, when they wheel Mum into the dorm, she manages to smile. A nurse reports that all has gone well. The operation was successful.

*

Efforts to get Mum to her feet over the next few days are met with resistance. It's as if she's forgotten what to do with her legs. She looks delirious, vacant.

There is a conversation in the corridor with a doctor. She asks if we think she will benefit from rehab; what we believe might be a realistic outcome. She gently suggests that should Mum get up, she would likely need the aid of a walker.

I respond by saying that Mum is no doubt still in shock following the fall and surgery. I believe that given time and support, she might walk again, albeit with a walker. I tell her that Mum has a very strong spirit, that she is very resilient. The doctor raises her eyebrow at the use of the word 'spirit' – it's about as non-medical as it gets – but she nods, agrees to start the ball rolling for admission to a nearby rehabilitation hospital.

Later that afternoon, there are more decisions to be made as I pull out of the hospital car park and another doctor calls – she talks me through the pros and cons of increasing Mum's aspirin dose to reduce the chance of further strokes. She explains that this increases the risk of bleeding if she gets a cut or falls. We talk about whether the benefits will outweigh the downsides. She patiently answers my questions. We agree that a higher aspirin dose will be prescribed.

Back at the hospital, Mum says she just wants to go home. But her list of ailments makes it seem unlikely. I explain that we are going to a hospital that will help her to walk, a bit like the one she went to after her stroke. She liked it there. She nods in understanding.

'Do you trust me, Mum?' This is always my go-to question when big decisions need to be made. I'm asking it more often these days.

'*Nai.*' Yes.

Not for the first time, I am both grateful and trepidatious that Mum has so much faith in me. I don't want to fail her.

The next day, Mum is transferred to a rehabilitation ward at the former Heidelberg Repatriation Hospital. Over the course of its 140-year history, the hospital has housed 'incurables' with tuberculosis and cancer. It served as a military hospital during the '40s. Its peeling covered walkways, disused outbuildings and a bomb shelter flank the grounds like maimed soldiers. Near the entrance to the main building, stained-glass windows with black-and-white images of war set against brightly coloured glass sharply contrast the sun-faded grounds. Inside, the hallway is lined with black-and-white photos of gaunt soldiers gathered around a table, stern-looking matrons in starched uniforms.

Mum and I have visited patients here several times: Mum's sister Voula, and Katina, a family friend from Mum's village. Katina was in a room with another Greek woman and a Greek priest, all of whom were introduced to us. Banter flowed back and forth across the beds. Katina started singing in Greek, surprising us with her melodic voice. The song's lyrical notes evoked another time and place – olive groves, clear blue seas, whitewashed walls. As Katina sang, I'd imagined my Mum and her as girls, laughing, their future full of possibility.

Mum is put in a room with three elderly men. A nurse takes her vitals, and I answer more questions. While the nurses change Mum and take out the intravenous canula in her hand, a white-haired lanky chap called Bob tells me he is going to live with his son and his daughter-in-law when he gets well. At the end of visiting hours, I put the nurse call button in Mum's hands, explaining again how to use it. Mum nods but looks at it blankly. I dawdle at the door, think how small and vulnerable she looks in the bed. How will she tell the nurses what she needs? How will they understand her? And how will she feel among all these men?

'Don't worry, love. We'll call the nurses if she needs anything,' Bob says, sending me off with a reassuring nod.

When I arrive early the next day, Mum's bed is empty, and her things are missing from the cupboard. I stifle an urge to panic. A nurse in the corridor informs me that Mum has been moved because she wouldn't let the other patients sleep. Staff were unable to work out what she wanted. She was a bit *disruptive*. I'm surprised. My mother has never disrupted anything in her life.

She leads me to a room opposite the nurse's station, which Mum has all to herself. When I ask Mum what happened last night, she mumbles about a man wanting to steal her things. She doesn't seem distressed, just confused. *It's okay Mum. You're in hospital. See, your things are here ...* She looks at me blankly. I hold her hand, hoping that touch will convey what words can't.

A petite, fast-moving woman with sharp features comes in. I gather she is the unit manager. We met her last night when she bundled up to me in the common area where I was sharing a snack with Mum. She'd told me that my mask needed to be kept on *at all times* because patients were *vulnerable*. And *please* remember to adhere to visiting hours.

In a complete about-face she now explains that I'm allowed to stay with Mum whenever I like, visit outside of hours if need be. I can even sleep over. She repeats that they moved Mum because she was *disruptive*. Her voice gives away that she thinks Mum is going to be one of those *difficult patients* that need to be *managed*. It feels like we've stepped back into one of the photos with stiff-backed matrons in starched caps lining the corridor walls downstairs. *I need to maintain order in the ranks. Anyone who steps out of line will be brought to task.*

In the last 72 hours, Mum has fallen, had surgery, been in a room with strange men and had nurses waking her at odd hours. She has dementia and can barely be understood in Greek, much less English. She is likely delirious. It stands to reason why she might be acting out in the way she was. I want to say, *My mother is the least difficult person you are likely to meet. She is just expressing her needs any way she can. At least she still has a bit of fight in her.* But I bite my tongue. Mum has her own room, and I have free rein to visit whenever I want. This must be a win in a system with such limited resources. Even if I can't be here, I know others can be – my brother, cousins, family friends. We have wrestled back some control.

*

The next day, Mum has her first session of physiotherapy. Dennis comes in and we look on as the physiotherapist tries to get Mum to stand. We interpret instructions, try to jolly her along with words of encouragement. She is willing to be supported by two people by her side but seems to have forgotten what to do with her legs. I sense her fear. Fear of pain, fear of falling. I convey this to the physiotherapist.

The following day, the physiotherapist places a supportive rail in front of Mum, assures her that the bed is behind her for support, that she needn't be scared. Still, Mum can't stand. She looks bewildered. For the first time, my faith in Mum's spirit, in her resilience in the face of adversity, falters. Perhaps her fear is too great, her dementia simply too far gone for her brain to tell her legs what to do? This is yet another downward step we will need to get our heads around.

A few days later, the physiotherapist stops me in the corridor, where I'm on the way to a meeting with a social worker. He doesn't think there is any point in continuing with therapy. Various attempts to get Mum to her feet have led nowhere. She is not responding at all. Perhaps when things settle, she will slowly try to get up by herself…

In the meeting with the social worker, we talk about the next steps. I say that the option for Mum to go back home, to live with my brother or to move in with my family and I, is simply not feasible. This has been months coming, and the decision would appear to have been taken out of our hands – how can we possibly take Mum back home when she needs two people to lift and turn her, when she is fully incontinent and when the symptoms of her dementia are now so much more challenging?

Humanity

The social worker hands me a folder which contains a list of aged care homes, a stack of government-generated information sheets on aged care and Mum's residential care code printed in large font on a single piece of paper. She explains the financial aspects of residential care. There is a daily fee, which everyone pays. This is set at 85% of the aged care pension, and is paid directly to the home. There may be care and accommodation costs which can be paid monthly, or through something called the RAD – a refundable accommodation deposit. This is a lump sum payment to the home. Each home sets its own RAD, which can range from a few hundred thousand dollars for very basic accommodation, to many hundreds of thousands for upmarket or exclusive facilities.

I already know from the Australian Government My Aged Care website that the fees will depend on Mum's income and assets, along with the level of care she requires and the home we choose. There is a fee estimate calculator on their site. We will need to fill in a form with Services Australia to get a means assessment. It's best to do this before she enters care. I make a note to push this task to the top of the priority list.

The hospital requires us to demonstrate that we have Mum on three waiting lists for care. A date for discharge is set for two weeks from now. If a home isn't found, we have the option to transfer Mum to a geriatric facility in a nearby suburb, which sounds to me like a no-man's land for elderly people with nowhere else to go. The subtext is clear. *We can't help her here anymore. We need her bed for someone who* can *be rehabilitated.*

I don't want to move Mum any more than is necessary. She's already been through enough. I tell the social worker that I'd visited several residential care homes over the summer, will get on the phone to the most promising ones to see which has a place for Mum.

On the way out, my godsister Gina rings, and the tears that have been threatening all morning finally flow. I tell Gina Mum won't walk again, that she is going to go into care. She says she is cooking a *pastichio*, a pasta bake, for her son, but she will switch off her oven and meet me in 20 minutes. When she arrives, I wet her shoulder with my tears, nose running.

She leads me to a café and we talk about Mum and the decline in her health; about us as children sitting cross-legged on the floor eating fish and chips at our shop, which is not more than a few kilometres away from here; of Mum working in Gina's mother's factory; of Gina's mum being there when I found out that Dad was dying, and my crying on *her* shoulder too. When I'm all cried out, and our shared memories thoroughly mined, I tell her how grateful I am – and that she should really get back to her *pastichio*.

*

In between managing hospital visits, home and work, a friend and I find time to go for a walk. Though she's having many of her own troubles – treatment for breast cancer, an elderly mother who is experiencing excruciating back pain, and a sick husband – she listens patiently. I talk about what has happened to Mum and about plans to get her into residential care. Despite all the events of the previous week, I feel a sense of relief. At least the responsibility for Mum's care has been taken out of our hands. At least now we know she will be safe. Though we will still need to be on top of things, still need to keep an eye on Mum, others will be available 24/7 to manage her care.

Early the next morning, the phone rings. Experience tells me that early-morning and late-night calls rarely signal good news.

'Chrisoula had a fall in the night. She's okay. We've been monitoring her …'

How can Mum, who can barely turn in her bed, have possibly fallen?

'She'll go in for a CT head scan this morning to check for a concussion. It's standard procedure after a fall …'

The voice on the other end of the phone responds to my questions in reassuring tones. *No one saw her fall. No, the rail wasn't up. She landed on the side of her broken hip.*

An hour later, I'm at the hospital. Mum is resting in bed. She looks fine. I ask her if she remembers falling last night. She can't quite articulate what happened. It sounds like she was trying to go to the toilet, or to leave the hospital. She looks a bit sheepish.

I stand to the side when nurses come in to change her before she goes down for the scan. She groans more loudly than usual, sounds like she is in pain. *A lot of pain.* When the intern comes in, I tell him that Mum seems to be in a lot more pain than usual.

'Please can you arrange for an x-ray?'

'I would need to get the registrar to order it …'

He is polite, but he looks like he wishes I wasn't asking for this. I know my mother well enough to know that something has changed. And it seems to me that the logical thing to do after a fall is to check if there's been a break. I meet his gaze evenly.

'Mum's not a complainer. Even when she broke her hip, she didn't let on that she was in pain. Something's wrong …'

By the time I accompany Mum down to the imaging department, an x-ray has been ordered along with the head scan. Soon after we come back up to the ward, the results are in. *A fracture in the greater trochanter.* Someone at the desk explains that this is another bone of the hip, very close to the first fracture in the neck of the femur. The surgery site doesn't appear to have been impacted.

I'm trying to find out what this means for Mum – if she will need more surgery, whether it will further affect her chances of walking again, how much pain it is likely to cause her – when the unit manager bundles into the room. I look at her expectantly, think she's here to talk about Mum's fall, but she doesn't meet my eyes. She's here to ask the nurse whether she's free to work during the long weekend a week from now.

Humanity

A moment later, I'm staring at her retreating back, incredulous. How can she not even have *acknowledged* Mum's fall?

*

'I'm so angry. They should have had the rails up. Or put the bed down low. She's got dementia for fuck's sake, of course she's going to try to get out of bed.' My cousin Dim lets rip on the other end of the phone after my message that Mum's fall has led to a new fracture.

'I'm angry too, Dim.' I look at Mum, try to keep my voice low so as not to upset her. 'But it's happened now, and there's no going back …'

'She's going to be in *so much* pain. I should have said something about lowering the bed when I was there last. I'm kicking myself now.'

I too question whether this could have been avoided. And if it happened to Mum, it can happen to someone else. While it's too late for Mum, I contemplate whether complaining will help to avoid it in future. But what if putting in a formal complaint means that Mum's care is compromised? And do I have the mental energy needed? Like Mum, I hate complaining, making a fuss. Mum's need to speak kindly, to be polite, has been ingrained in me. But she is also wily, a survivor, and I need to channel that now.

I do it in the best way I know how: subversively. When I casually question why the rail was down, a nurse explains that dementia patients have further to fall if they climb over a rail. Another says that low beds can be overwhelming and scary for dementia patients, especially as they are sharing with three others whose beds are looming over them. Another tells me that Mum didn't call out after her fall. That when someone came into the room, Mum waved at them from the floor, ever polite. I fossick for morsels of information that might help me build a picture, feel a bit sorry for the nurses who are cornered into answering my questions.

On the Monday after the fall, I have a brief conversation with an orthopaedic doctor, who explains that Mum will be unable to bear weight on her legs for six weeks as a result of the break. Stronger painkillers have been prescribed. The bed has been lowered and crash mats have been put in place. Any visitors are instructed to ask nurses to make sure the bed is lowered after a visit has ended.

As the days pass, I feel more and more dismayed as Mum becomes less coherent, her face grimacing in pain when staff change her. After strong pain medication is administered, she falls into a deep sleep. When she wakes up, she looks off into the distance, barely registers that I'm there, picks at her food. She is on laxatives to combat the constipating effects of the strong opioids she is now on and needs to be changed more often, causing her more distress. I sit in the white-walled room, feeling increasingly angry that things have gone seriously downhill since she fell. I turn my distress and lack of agency inwards.

It tastes bitter, feels dark. I berate myself that I can't properly advocate for my mother at her time of greatest need.

I don't know who to talk to. I consider speaking to the unit manager. I imagine myself saying to her, *I'm angry that this happened. I wonder if it could have been avoided. It's too late for Mum, but I don't want it to happen to others.* What I would like her to say is this: *I am sorry that this happened. We too don't want it to happen to other patients. We are looking into how we might avoid it in future.* But the cynic in me envisages a very different scenario. The nurse manager would get defensive and say the same things that the nurses have told me. I would get more frustrated, perhaps think about making a formal complaint. But that's something that requires time and energy, which I simply don't have. My focus is squarely on Mum, and there is no room for anything else right now.

A few days later, I'm surprised and pleased when several people come into the room in quick succession to provide an update on Mum – the physio, the social worker, the doctor. The physio explains that with this new break, the main implication is that Mum will need to use a walker for six weeks if she gets up again. *If* she gets up again. That's now even more unlikely. He says it is safe to get her to sit up in the wheelchair, okay to take her outside when she is feeling up to it. I tell the social worker about the lack of places available in the care homes we have chosen. For Mum to stay here, she reminds me that we only need to show we have approached three facilities. The doctor talks about trying slow-release pain meds to combat the peaks and troughs of Mum's pain. She explains that the eventual aim of treatment will be to wean her off strong pain medication, and that she will become more lucid as a result. I ask her the one question that's been plaguing me.

'Is Mum close to dying?' I look towards Mum, who lies semi-comatose on the bed.

Her answer is considered. 'It's a question your cousin alluded to when she visited this morning. While we can't say how long someone will live, once we properly manage her pain, she'll be okay for discharge to residential care.'

It's as if a big weight has been lifted off my shoulders. While the fall was unfortunate, we can now work towards getting Mum out of here.

That afternoon, when my cousin Kathy rings, I explain the latest developments to her, telling her I'm pleasantly surprised that so many people took the time to speak to me today.

'Well, so they should. I came in this morning and gave them a piece of my mind, didn't I? I said to them, "Look at my aunty. Just look at her. She looks like she's dying. She came here to get better, but she's much worse off than when she came in because she fell. What are you doing about it?!"'

*

Over the next few weeks, Mum's pain starts to be better managed, and she becomes a bit more lucid. We get into a routine of sorts. On sunny days, we sit in the garden and eat eggs and grapes and custard: food I know she likes, offered in a bid to tempt her to eat. The days when she manages to laugh, or responds to a conversation with understanding, are like a gift. I tell her repeatedly that I love her.

The restrictions ease up a little so that four people are now able to visit each day. Between our family, Dennis, my cousins and family friends, Mum has twice-daily visitors almost every day. George organises meals and keeps the wheels of our home oiled and turning so that I can continue to work and see Mum each day. He and the kids are quick with firm hugs when I burst into tears after particularly challenging visits. Friends and family check in regularly to ask how we are going. Surrounded by all this support, I find reserves of energy I didn't know I had. But in the hospital room, day in, day out, I can't help feeling isolated. I look forward to the day when we will be able to leave the room's faded walls.

I make regular phone calls and send emails to Greek care homes from my car, checking to see availabilities, but there is nothing. When it's clear that we are unlikely to get into our preferred Greek facilities, I extend the search, ask for recommendations to see if there are other suitable facilities in suburbs with a high Greek population. I still feel committed to Mum hearing familiar language around her, hope that this will help make the stay in a care home less difficult. Though my father-in-law's home is an excellent facility, and we consider placing Mum there, there isn't a single Greek speaker there, and it's too far on the other side of town for family to visit regularly. I get my hands on a list from a former carer and call each place to see what is available. Some say there are no places, others don't return my calls.

I sit on the phone with Centrelink and My Aged Care for hours to find out if my brother, who has always lived with Mum and has up until recently been on a disability pension, is considered a 'protected person'. If he is, Mum's home will not be counted as an asset. This will impact the cost of her care, which is likely to be considerable. The hold music gets on my nerves, and there are times when I want to throw the phone across the room. I am asked to fill out forms about Dennis's and Mum's financial situation, each requiring several pieces of supporting evidence. Each time, I am asked to verify my identity, prove why I, and not Mum or Dennis, am calling. I think back to Jean's Kittson's advice: get professional help if you can afford it – and keep a notebook. I approach a financial counsellor who specialises in aged care, but decide not to go ahead with their help as I have already done most of the leg work myself. The enduring power of attorney documents are getting a workout as I send them across to various people to verify my right to act on Mum's behalf. It feels like we filled them out a lifetime ago.

After a month of visiting and sitting with Mum every day, I take a day off to give our home a good clean, to glean back some control. Dennis rings, says Mum is asking for me. Mum rarely asks for anything, and so I go back to be with her.

I think back to the time she first had her stroke, where she wasn't yet able to cobble together any decipherable words, could barely stand. Still, she felt she had come off lightly – the Greek man in the bed across from her had had a bigger stroke. His wife came to talk to Mum, held her hand as they cried together. A few days later, when she found out the man had been moved to a private room because he was dying, Mum insisted on getting up to pay her respects to the family. Even in her grimmest hour, Mum wanted to help ease the family's pain. I want to do the same for her now.

Finally, I come across a home that has a bed for Mum. It's Friday afternoon when I ring to make enquiries. The client services manager asks if I am free to come in right away. On the tour, the home looks promising – it is clean, and I meet several Greek residents as we make our way around the facility. I'm concerned that most of the rooms are shared, but the client services officer assures me that roommates generally enjoy the company and often become friends. Mum would be in with a Greek lady, who isn't in her room when I visit. My first impressions are favourable, and I feel the pressing need to get Mum out of hospital and settled. The client services officer tells me to ring her over the weekend if we have questions. That we need to let her know promptly if we want to take the room, as she has had several people in today. I discuss it with my brother, check the home's credentials on the My Aged

Care website and make the call on the Monday morning. I'm relieved when we set a date for admission. We can finally leave the white hospital room.

*

As our discharge date comes around, I organise flowers and chocolates for the hospital staff. While I've been frustrated and upset at the turn of events, staff on the ground have been unfailingly kind and diligent. It's the least I can do to say thank you. I've listened to the banter between the nurses, gauged something of their personalities and interests over our six-week stay here. I marvel once again at how they do such a challenging job each day. Those who have cared for Mum drop in to say she has been a joy to look after, to wish her luck, to give her a hug.

The discharge day arrives, and while we wait for the patient transport to come, Mum's bag of clothes and a few toiletries neatly packed beside us, Mum dozes, her mouth open. Her face is pale, her cheeks sunken. It's hard to believe that last month she was shuffling around her home, still able to walk around the block, able to make jokes.

Mum stirs, asks what is happening. I remind her that we are leaving today, moving to a new place. I avoid using the phrase *gerokomeio*, care home, but I'm quite sure she knows what I mean. I say with forced cheerfulness that she will have the company of other Greek women, that she won't be alone.

'*Pame spiti?*' Are we going home?

'We can't go home, Mamma. You are too sick. I'm sorry.'

We've had this conversation before, but it's like she's hearing it for the first time. She looks to the wall, and I look at my hands. I have no words to make this better.

*

Shortly after, the cleaner comes in and starts cleaning around us. I can't help but think that no matter how many times she passes her mop over the scratched linoleum, the rubberised lines made by so many commodes, wheelchairs, and beds on castors won't shift. The grey patches and layers of peeling paint on the walls and ceiling suggest the room might have been part of the original wing of this former military hospital. Mum is feasibly one of thousands of patients who have been cared for here. What if the walls were like a sea sponge – porous, living – able to soak up something of the whispered conversations, the moans in the night, the cries of pain? What might all this accumulated suffering look like? I imagine vapours rising from the plaster, ghostly forms walking the hallways at night.

My thinking is morbid and jaded. It disturbs me. I've felt these walls closing in around me these past weeks. Images of Mum's feet trembling in pain as she is lifted into a harness, her quietly putting up with the indignity of being changed and turned, showered and toileted, plague my dreams at night. I wake consistently at 4 each morning, unable to get back to sleep.

I'm startled out of my dark musings: the patient transport is here.

As Mum is wheeled out of the room, I happen to stand beside the unit manager in the corridor. She lets on that because of Mum's fall, they have had to set up new protocols for their unit. That any dementia patients admitted are to be put in low beds with crash mats. She shares the information with me begrudgingly, doesn't meet my eyes. It's clear the process has inconvenienced her. I am astounded that we are having this conversation weeks after Mum fell.

I stare at her, force her to meet my eyes. I tell her that if anything good has come out of this difficult scenario that has caused *Mum* so much pain, it is that it has led to a change that might help others who are equally *vulnerable*. Her eyes flit away, but I know she's heard what I have to say. It's enough for now.

As Mum is wheeled out, I look back to see that the bed is already being stripped, that fresh linen has been brought in. Someone new will make more buff marks, leave more stains. I don't know what we've left of ourselves in the room's white walls, but there's no time to dwell on that anymore. We need to move on.

GIFT #8

Persistence

I will act when you need me to

March 2023

Mum is sitting up in her new bed. The client services officer is making a fuss of her, asking if she wants ice cream. When Mum nods, she goes off to get the events coordinator – and there is lots of fanfare as a retro-looking peddle cart is pushed down the corridor and parked outside Mum's door. I have a flashback of the Mr Whippy van that used to come up the street in Collingwood on Saturday afternoons, its tinny music making Dennis and I salivate like Pavlov's dog. We would beg Mum for coins, and more often than not, she would oblige us so we could run down the street for ice cream.

The cart is parked in front of the little sink plastered with handwashing signs, sanitising soaps and lotions. The events coordinator makes small talk as she scoops up the ice cream – I learn that she's one of two Greek-speaking staff in this home of more than 120 residents, who mostly hail from southern Europe. The other Greek speaker is the cleaner. The events coordinator talks about how hard it is to find staff that speak the languages of the older Greek and Italian immigrants that emigrated in the '50s and '60s.

Persistence

While we are talking, my cousin Dim rings to find out how the transfer went. I tell her Mum is eating ice cream. She says she likes this place already, is pleased that Mum is settling in.

In the early evening, Mum's new roommate is wheeled into the room and introductions made. When the worker leaves, Mum's roommate asks her to repeat her name. She is irritated when Mum can't respond, and I explain that Mum has trouble communicating. When I state Mum's name, several times as she tells me she is hard of hearing, she starts repeating it in different variations in a singsong voice: *Tsintziras, Tzitzikas, Mitzikas, Bitzikas,* as if she is teasing the new girl on the school ground. Mum looks bewildered. I sit between the two women, wondering where this will go. Finally, when neither of us respond, Mum's roommate switches on her television and looks away from us. I quietly pull the curtain across the two beds and turn my attention back to Mum. Somehow, I don't think a friendship is going to form here.

*

Over coming days there are the morning ablutions, breakfast served in bed, activities like bingo and balloon football, and lunch in the dining room. I doubt Mum will get much out of the activities, but it's good to know there are some distractions. That evening, there are a few phone calls back and forth between the nurse and myself to sort out some confusion around Mum's drugs. I've been given a wad of forms to fill out. There are new systems and staff to get used to.

Still, as the week comes to an end, Mum seems settled. Her roommate doesn't appear to spend much time in the room, and I haven't seen a repeat of the first night's behaviour.

George comes in to visit, and we can't help comparing the home to his dad's: Mum's section is locked away from the main area, and the dining area is often eerily quiet outside of mealtimes. He finds it disconcerting when, out of the corner of his eye, he sees two staff bring in an agitated resident. Afterwards, he whispers to me that they were rough when seating him down. He's never seen anything like that at his dad's home. I hear what he is saying, but part of me just wants to get on with it, to push through. *We are finally here now after our terrible experience at the hospital. We have to make this work.*

Emmanuel and Dolores visit on separate occasions. Dolores blow-dries Mum's hair, and I take a video for posterity: I'm all too aware that the remaining opportunities to record Mum with her grandchildren are getting fewer and fewer. I feel awkward about it, have been hesitant these past weeks to photograph Mum looking so compromised.

When Emmanuel visits after work, he sits by Mum's bed and holds her hand, looks into her eyes. Though he doesn't speak much Greek, the bond with his grandmother has always been strong. She seems to understand him, always accepted him unconditionally. Though he towers over her, his gestures are gentle, loving. It saddens me to see him in such robust good health compared to Mum, who looks like a diminutive, washed-out version of her former self on the white bed.

On the way out, I tell Emmanuel how much it means to Yiayia that he is here. I know he doesn't like visiting residential care homes. As I lead him out to the foyer, I ask him what he thinks of this home.

He shrugs, looks up past the chandeliers and plush seating, down the corridor where a cacophony of voices and raucous activity can be heard. A resident tries to edge past him, her walker bashing at the home's glass doors. A staff member leads her away.

'Oh, Mum, they're all the same. Someone's always screaming, and someone's always trying to get out.'

*

Mum's face contorts with discomfort, but she tries to compose herself to say goodbye, to send my brother and me off. Her carer has her plastic gloves on, and the hoist is out – it's finally Mum's turn to be changed and put to bed.

Mum's had a good morning. She was sitting up in her wheelchair when we arrived, showered and dressed, hair slicked back and television on. She had colour in her cheeks. Her roommate was napping in her wheelchair. Mum was pleased to see us after her initial confusion – my brother and I have been taking it in shifts to visit, but today we have come in together. I put my bag down, give her a kiss through my mask. Dennis does the same. I take out the *kourabiethes*, sugar-dusted shortbreads, that I made that morning, remind her it is nearly Greek Easter. That she will be coming to our house on Sunday.

'How will I know … how …?'

'I have organised everything. A taxi will come to get you. I'll be with you all the time.'

I explain that she needn't worry about a thing, that she doesn't have to think about the when or what of it all. Just that we are gathering at our house for lunch. She nods, reassured.

'It's sunny outside. Do you want to go for a walk?'

'Why not?' she says. She's been in the new care home for two weeks, and apart from a few laps around the corridors and into the courtyard, she hasn't been out. I place a blanket on her lap, and we make our way down the corridor. The staff are preparing for lunch, placing trays on tiered trolleys. The cleaner is making his way around each room, going back and forth with his own trolley. The dining room, usually bustling with activity, is silent. There has been a gastro outbreak and a case of Covid in one of the downstairs wings, and residents are all in their rooms. We walk past the view, where you might just see the Dandenong Ranges if you lean your head just so. Dennis pushes the wheelchair, and I make small talk with Mum about the weather, about the kids, about what's in our garden. At the nurse's station, a carer waves us off, mentions that Mum had a good breakfast. I'm glad, because her appetite has been erratic at best. I clock his name on his name badge, make an effort to use it to thank him. Finally, we make our way outside.

Mum looks around with interest. I tell her again what suburb we are in, that there is a school next door. She looks at the houses curiously, recognises an olive tree, states what it is clearly. When I express my surprise and delight, she says, 'Well, of course I know what it is. I grew up with it.' Her ability to articulate her thoughts and use the right words to name things is getting more and more erratic. It's getting harder to understand her, even in Greek. I joke that she was born in the 'time of the olive harvest' in Greece. Her birthdate was never recorded.

On the way back, we stop to let her take in the façade of the care home. I look at her carefully, and she doesn't appear distressed to be returning. This makes me glad – another sign that she is settling in as well as can be expected.

Back in her room, a resident comes in, sits on Mum's bed. She holds Dennis's hand, engages him in a conversation that doesn't always make sense. It becomes clear she is looking for a sibling long dead. Mum looks on, her eyes saying, *What is she doing here?* A carer comes along, takes the resident by the elbow and leads her out. She clings to Dennis's hand as long as possible.

A food tray is delivered – today there is soup, moussaka, halva and custard. The meal looks appetising, but Mum is not excited. She seems to have forgotten how to feed herself over the past few weeks since being in hospital, has lost her appetite. I feed her soup, which is easy to eat. She has a few spoonfuls of eggplant, pulls a face. I feed her some halva, which she seems to like.

'Remember when we used to make halva?'

She nods. '*Hrmph*, now I can't do anything …'

It's true. The losses have been so numerous in the past few months. She had wished to die in her own home. To die in her own bed. But here we are. Now she has broken her hip, she can no longer feed herself, go to the toilet, walk or properly express what she needs. The opportunity to die in her own bed has become very slim. The thought fills me with an overwhelming sadness. I push it down, make small talk, busy myself trying to cajole her to eat just one more spoonful of halva.

Soon after, Mum soils herself, as she often does after lunch. I press the button for a carer to come. A few minutes in, the carer comes in to turn the call button off. She says that they are still in the lunchtime service, and that she will be back in five or ten minutes. When I explain to Mum, she nods. She can wait.

Twenty minutes later, Mum becomes agitated. She is uncomfortable. I find another carer, and she tells me there are no staff available at the moment – two staff are needed to hoist mum. Mum's roommate presses her button and starts to wriggle in her chair. When no one comes, she calls out loudly that she needs to be taken to the toilet. She looks to us, and I'm reminded of something she said when we first arrived. That in her village, there is a saying: 'Those who don't scream get buried alive.'

Persistence

The cleaner, who is passing by, tells her that someone will clean her up if she soils herself, that's what's she paying for, and to please be patient. But she doesn't do patience well, and she starts to call out at the top of her voice. A carer comes in, and then soon after, another. They take her into the toilet, and she swears some more, calls out. Mum looks on, trying to lift her hips off her chair. It will be another 20 minutes before her neighbour's toileting needs are taken care of. Mum's discomfort escalates. She looks to me, implores me with her eyes to do something. When one of the carers comes out, and the other makes his way down the corridor with the hoist, I panic. Perhaps they are off to attend to someone else. Someone who has a louder voice than us. If we have been waiting this long while I am here, agitating, how long does Mum wait when I am not here?

In this moment, I know I must act. I stand before the carer can leave the room again.

'Please, Mum has soiled herself. She has been waiting for a long time ...' I can't help but keep the frustration out of my voice.

'We need to get her a different hoist. We take it room by room after lunch. You saw how long it took to take her roommate to the toilet.'

Her tone is reassuring but firm. There's no doubt that this isn't the first time she has had to talk a resident's family down.

We pressed Mum's buzzer before her roommate, I want to say to her, retreating as she makes her way down the corridor. I feel like I'm back in the school room, and that the naughty kids are getting all the attention.

I understand there are staffing shortages. That carers are paid not nearly enough to clean faeces, feed residents, deal with abuse and racism day in and day out. In the two weeks I've been here, I've heard abuse hurled at the staff by residents in the corridors and in the dining room and in the bedrooms when I've walked past.

But still, this is *my mother*. My poor gentle mother, who has no voice, who's been sitting in her own faeces for nearly an hour now.

Finally, a staff member wheels in the hoist, and another joins her. They move to draw the curtain around Mum's bed. It's time for us to leave. We kiss Mum again, leaving her in the blue-gloved hands of the carer who will divest her of her sanitary nappy and put her to bed.

*

A few days later, the client services officer emails to see if we are happy to switch Mum from respite to permanent care. Though we are looking for a permanent arrangement, respite care has bought us some time before Mum has to start paying accommodation fees and enter into a permanent care contract. Importantly, it's given us a chance to see if we are happy with the home.

Persistence

Mum seems to have settled in as well as can be expected. She is surrounded by Greek-speaking residents, a few who have taken a shining to her and seem to look out for her. The food is acceptable. Dennis seems to be getting more used to the idea of Mum being in care, is getting to know some of the fellow residents.

There are some things I don't like: Mum's roommate screams when she doesn't get what she wants, and it's hard to tell how she is when she is alone with Mum. Still, she doesn't spend a lot of time in the room, is often out in the common areas. When she's in the room of an evening, she mostly watches television.

Another thing that grates on me, particularly after the intimacy of the hospital room where I stood just metres from Mum no matter what was being done to her, is that I'm not allowed to be in the room when Mum is getting changed. When I question this, I am told firmly that it's about privacy, and about space – there is very little room with two carers and Mum for someone else to be present. The discussion is shut down quickly. It doesn't appear to be negotiable.

I can't help but compare this quite large care home to the much smaller one that my father-in-law is in. Most of the carers at his home are familiar, and many staff have been there a long time. Visitors are greeted warmly, and snippets about how my father-in-law is, what he did, are shared openly.

At this home, the residents are over two floors, and there are several wings. It appears that carers move between the floors when needed. Even a few weeks in, I still haven't got a handle on who does what, and who is who, or even what Mum does most days. It's disconcerting.

Still, I'm relieved that Mum doesn't appear too distressed. I tell myself that it's a matter of time before we get to know people, the lay of the land. I write to the client services officer, tell her that we are keen for Mum to have her own room when it becomes available. She assures me that she will put us on a waiting list. I pop my head into her office a few days later, reiterate what I've said in the email.

'Yes, I will let you know when a single room becomes available.'

I ask her something that has been troubling me. 'Is her roommate safe? She's not likely to hurt Mum?'

The client services officer laughs. 'She's harmless. You don't have anything to worry about.'

I tell her that we are happy to move to permanent care. To please send me the contract for us to review and sign.

*

Dim and Kathy have been in to visit Mum on a few occasions, sometimes taking Mum's sister with them. After her initial enthusiasm with the ice cream cart, Dim is not exactly enamoured with the new home.

Over a few phone conversations, she outlines her concerns. People with dementia need peace and quiet –

Mum is too close to the door, appears unsettled every time unfamiliar people walk up and down. She notes that infection control is very difficult in a shared room. That the carers who come into the room don't introduce themselves as they should, don't seem particularly pleased to see that Mum has visitors. She and Kathy word their concerns carefully, try to curb their usual forward style, but the implication is clear: Mum deserves more.

I agree that the shared room isn't ideal. I find myself getting defensive. *It's taken me a long time to find this place. Mum is settling as well as can be expected. We're on a waiting list for a single room. Yes, of course Mum deserves more, the best, but this is the best we can do* right now.

Even as I speak these words, I understand their concerns. There are times when the care doesn't feel very personal. Staff sometimes don't look very confident or pleased to be working here. And I have to work hard to get information.

I've just completed the slew of forms involved in putting someone in care, only just started to get to know who does what. It's taken a long time to find a home, and I'm not wanting to uproot Mum again unless there is a very good reason to. I don't want to make any kneejerk decisions: my biggest fear is that I might jump out of the frying pan and into the fire.

*

The gastro outbreak that was downstairs has made its way to Mum's wing, and I can't visit her. I ring the home to see how she is. I am told she is doing fine. For the first time, I ask the carer to pass the phone to Mum so I can speak to her. She takes the phone to Mum, and all I can hear is, *Oh God, Oh God, Oh God …*

I try to tell Mum it's me, ask if she can hear me, whether she could pass the phone back to the carer … but she repeats the words over and over, and it's clear the carer is not in the room. Several minutes later, I hang up. I'm shocked and disturbed. I have never heard Mum like that. When I ring the home again, the line rings out. I ring later, and the carer tells me Mum is settled, sleeping soundly.

A few days later, the gastro outbreak is over, and we are allowed to visit again.

I walk past a room with two empty beds, the name tags gone from the wall outside, and another with one empty bed. I shudder. I imagine these residents have died following the outbreak.

Mum is sitting in the common area, facing the television. As always, she is glad to see me. I ask a carer how Mum is, whether she's been eating and sleeping.

'We're feeding her. I don't know about sleep. That was the last shift …' She looks a bit wary. It's not the first time I've seen this look, which seems to say, *Please don't ask me any questions.*

My cousins' concerns reverberate in my head: there is a conspicuous lack of warmth here.

Persistence

The glossy brochure I was given on the tour explains who does what and the uniforms they wear: the personal carers, the nurses, the clinical coordinator and the ancillary staff. But on the ground, it's hard to get my bearings, to tell who does what. You can't always see carers' name badges, and apart from one or two, they don't seem to know Mum very well. The nurses' station is often unattended, and when I enter, staff avert their eyes. Staff are masked, and it's hard to make connections: I can't even begin to think how Mum feels about this. Still, I've gotten to know a few people, and I feel at least there are some who will answer any questions I have about Mum's wellbeing. I cling to them like a lifeline.

In a subsequent visit, I notice one of the single rooms becomes available, but before I can speak to the client services officer, a new resident has been placed within. They won't stop screaming, wandering the hallways asking for help, to be let out, grasping at Dennis and I when we walk past.

The empty rooms following the gastro outbreak have irked me: I wonder about how infection is controlled in a place where the beds are so close to each other. I email the client services manager again about a single room, and she repeats briefly: 'When it becomes available.' But with so few single rooms in this home, I can't imagine we are high on the priority list.

*

Twelve Golden Gifts

I'm sitting with Mum in the dining area, spooning food into her mouth. The other residents have finished their meals, and the carers are tidying up the last of the dinner things. It's raucous; a spat breaks out, there is screaming coming from a room up the hall, and there's the loud clank of dishes being wiped down and stacked into the dishwasher. I can see the two carers on the floor hesitant to approach the feuding residents. They look a little out of their depth.

During the week, I'd gotten a call that Mum had fallen out of her wheelchair. The fall had happened in the dining area, was not sighted by staff. I'd asked questions to glean what might have happened. Had the wheelchair been found tipped over? *No.* Where was she found? *At the front of the wheelchair.* I have noticed that when she gets tired, or has been sitting too long, her body slides forward, but it's a stretch to think how she could slide out if her leg supports were up. I feel ill on hearing the news. How many more indignities and challenges must my poor mother face?

The worker had told me they were monitoring Mum, that she didn't appear to be in pain. They had said they would ring me if anything changed. The information was delivered briefly, and the tone didn't invite questions. I can't help comparing this response to those that George gets after any falls his father has had. George's dad is mobile, but very frail, and has had quite a few falls when moving around in his room. The information the home provides after such falls is very forthcoming – with details about how he will be monitored and how often. It is distressing for all when someone falls, and they always take such incidents seriously.

When I'd gone in shortly after, Mum remembered nothing about falling. When she was being changed, I'd listened outside her door for new sounds of discomfort, but there were none. Later, I'd ran my hands over her arms and legs, asked her if she felt pain anywhere, checked for bruising. She did not, and there were no marks on her skin. Still, I was perturbed. How long was she sitting in her wheelchair unobserved?

After the incident, the legs of her wheelchair were adjusted to avoid something like this happening again. But still, as I spoon another mouthful of soft food into Mum's mouth, I feel a shift.

Over the past two months, I've tried my best to work out how to navigate this system to get Mum decent care. But as time has gone on, instead of my faith in the home growing, it's eroding. It feels like it's just a matter of time before something terrible happens. It's time to start looking for a new home.

*

Don't cry, don't cry. Think of something else. You can't help Mum if you're crying.

I'm sitting in the GP's waiting room one evening. This is the first time I've come here without Mum, and the empty waiting room makes me feel lonely. Alone. But I talk myself down before the tears can start. *You're here to help Mum. Pull yourself together.*

This most recent search for aged care homes started in earnest at the My Aged Care site. I'd pored over homes at night, methodically looking at quality, staffing, compliance. I'd cross-referenced ratings, which are based on percentages of reported falls, unexplained weight loss, drug use to control residents' behaviour, and how many staffing minutes were allocated per resident. My logical, ordered brain tries to clasp desperately at things I can understand – statistics, tables – the maths of care. Now I've given up on exclusively Greek homes, the list of options is endless.

I've used the trusty Jean Kittson guide on what to look for in an aged care home, but the list is mind-boggling. This assumes a perfect world where there is bed availability. I've tried to make a sensible shortlist based on things that are important to us – good care, decent proximity to Mum's home, and a medium-sized home with sound infrastructure, but not so big as to be impersonal.

I'd made several phone calls to visit those on my shortlist. Some got back, others didn't. When I visited, I would park outside, get my list of questions and notes out. *How could they help Mum communicate her needs? How did they communicate with family? Would Mum be in a dementia-specific ward?*

The few I'd seen during the week had reminded me of hotels. There were those with cavernous hallways and closed doors, mood lighting and floral arrangements, libraries and mirrored entry ways. Some hit you with strong smells of sickly cleaning fluid as soon as you walked in. The client services officers would walk me through and hand over packs with price lists and glossy brochures. I'd go back into the car, jot down impressions with a heavy heart. Logic and order had gone out the window. Instinct kicked in. *This is not the one.*

I couldn't visualise Mum in these places. She needs quiet, but she also needs some stimulation and warmth. Perhaps a few Greek voices. A bit of life. But above all, good care. Perhaps I was looking for something that wasn't quite possible, trying to replicate her home, her family. Somewhere where they could see past the ageing body and into her cheeky eyes, draw a chuckle. It was getting hard for me to do these things, much less a carer who had a busy schedule of residents to bathe and change. I know I need to curb my expectations, deal with my own grief.

When the doctor calls me in, he asks after Mum. I summarise the past three months – Mum's fall, rehabilitation, her going into care. He asks how I am, and I try to hold back tears. A few escape.

'Please don't ask, John, because I will *really* cry.' I smile wryly.

He tells me that we had gone above and beyond in caring for Mum, done more than most would do. That our story is one he hears over and over in his practice: trying to care for someone with dementia at home, with all the escalating perils, gets harder and harder. The falls, the wandering at night, the incontinence. That often his patients did not want to go into care.

'I've heard this story so many times, Spiri. Dementia is a cruel disease. You lose your loved one twice. You lose them mentally, and then you lose them physically, when their body goes. And it can go on and on – it's such a long goodbye.'

What he says makes complete sense.

I lurch onto the business at hand.

'Mum's in care, but we're not really happy. She's in a shared room. We chose the place because there were lots of Greek residents there, so that she could hear Greek voices around her, not feel so alienated. But it turns out that Greeks with dementia are particularly loud!' I pause. John smiles on cue at my lame joke. It's my way of gleaning back some control.

'We'd like to bring her closer to her house, make it easier to bring her home sometimes, and so that we can visit regularly. Can you recommend any homes where you have patients?'

John gets down to business, suggests a few aged care homes nearby. Most are already on my shortlist. When I tell him what we are looking for, he reminds me not to look for perfection. I realise I am still dragging my feet. In my heart, I still didn't want Mum to be in care, but that horse has bolted.

On leaving, I thank John for his compassion and skill in looking after Mum. Nearly cry again. I walk out into the night with my shortlist of care homes, ticks beside the ones that John has recommended.

Persistence

I think about Mum. How she has such faith in me. For her sake, I really want to get it right this time.

*

A few days later, I visit yet another care home, and I'm feeling optimistic that this might be the one. My online research is promising – it's a 15-minute drive from our home so regular visits will be easy, they employ the Montessori method to work with people with dementia, it's a good size, and it's run by the local council.

I struggle to find it on the sprawling grounds that houses several health and aged care units and buildings. There are various small car parks dotted on the complex. I finally find the building I'm after, do the RAT test and don the masks that are sitting on a table outside. I've lost count of how many RAT tests I've done over the past few months, barely bat an eye at sticking the white rod well into my nostrils. The reception area is small and packed with posters and pamphlets. *Aggression will not be tolerated. Stay Covid safe. How to make a complaint.* I look down the long hallway, try to make eye contact with someone to let them know I've arrived. A harried looking woman comes in, makes a phone call on my behalf and tells me that the woman I'm meeting for a tour is on her way.

The tour guide is efficient – we walk the circuit of the facility, and she gives me a well-rehearsed spiel. The food on the trolleys reminds me of the meals that Mum got in hospital – neatly compartmentalised and nutritionally balanced. The hallways are pleasant, the common rooms still quiet as carers get residents out of bed and showered. The rooms look onto well-tended green spaces. I tell the tour guide about Mum, and she walks me out of the facility to another area that has more specialised dementia care. This area has more beds, three locked units coming off a common space. She apologises – she can't show me one area because there are active cases of Covid.

As I walk back to my car, my shoulders slump. Throughout the tour, I couldn't help but shake off the hospital vibe. Lush as the gardens were, something Mum would love, this is not the one.

*

I try and keep my anxiety at bay with exercise whenever I can find a spare hour. Punch it out at boxing classes, dance it out at Zumba. I even try a few sessions of underwater rugby in a desperate bid to push myself out of my head and physically tire myself out so I can sleep, but I quickly realise you can't breathe under water, and that I don't have time to commit to getting over my fear. My time is spent in tightly packed parcels: visiting Mum, going to work, looking after our home. Thankfully, our kids are young adults now, and they are taking life in their stride. George is still visiting his parents three times a week, but there haven't been any major emergencies for a while. For this I am grateful.

I pick up a book in the middle of the night to still my thoughts, to escape from them. I go on walks with friends, where I tell them about my worries, and they tell me about theirs. I debrief with my husband in bed, and my daughter in the car, with my son as he wanders into the kitchen for a snack. Where once I spoke with Mum over the phone each day, now I speak with Dennis, talk about how Mum's going, how he is. I am lucky to be surrounded by so many people I can talk to. I try to lose myself, step outside of my head and into their lives. But it's a fine line. I don't want to burden those around me with my worries. I keep my kitchen bench clean and our house in order, grumble at the kids to pick up after themselves. I take pleasure in cooking a meal and sharing it around the table with George and the children, and their friends. This fills me up, calms me down. Pouring the words onto the page helps too. It feels as if I am untangling a sort of madness, making sense of it.

I know that Mum has had a long life, that it is only natural for it to wane. But I feel it intensely, this losing of my mother in bits. Her sadness. My responsibility to her. My guilt that perhaps I have not done enough, can never do enough to compensate for all that she has done for me. I keep reminding myself that I can only do what I can. I can't solve this. I can't control the trajectory of her disease. I can only control what I can offer. I think back to the prayer, 'Grant me the serenity to accept the things I cannot change ...' Still, still ... I know all this intellectually. But my heart screams: *Don't go. Keep being who you are. Don't suffer.*

*

'I love you, Maria!' I say, interrupting her mid-sentence and touching her knee, as if to bring the point home.

Since I've just met Maria, I can only imagine what she is thinking – who *is* this mad woman? She's a little taken aback, but she goes with it, bursts into laughter.

She's taken me for a tour around the aged care home where she works. Declaring my love of a saleswoman who I've spent an hour with is insane. But I'm guessing she's used to all sorts of behaviours.

I've found this home through an agency that links people to aged care homes. It was recommended by the coordinator of Mum's Home Care Package, who had used this service to find a home for her own father. To date, I had been hesitant to use such a service, as I was concerned about the cost and how I might find an unbiased one. I was assured, however, that the service was free for users, and that they did not have 'preferred' sites. After speaking with me about what we were looking for, the service had made a shortlist of three homes which had available beds. This is the first of these that I'm seeing.

This home has ticked several boxes even before I'd walked in the door. It was a good size with some 60 beds – not too big and not too small. It had a memory support area. At this stage, Mum doesn't need to be placed in a dementia unit as she is not mobile, and isn't aggressive or very disruptive. Still, the unit is there should her circumstances change. It means she can get more specialised care down the track if she needs it. And their Facebook page was full of frivolity – a puppeteer crooning '50s ballads, Greek Easter egg painting led by one of the residents, an Anzac Day commemorative service and a drumming workshop where one of the staff joined in passionately. As I'd driven up to the door, I'd said a little prayer. *Please let this be the one.*

The administration area was busy with movement when I'd walked in. The manager's door was open, and a staff member appeared to have dropped in. They walk out smiling. A resident was hurrying out to the bus for an excursion. I wasn't the only one waiting for a tour. There is a family grappling with the check-in monitor: there's a bewildered-looking man leaning over his walker; a fit-looking woman with coiffed hair; and an adult daughter perhaps, whose face was set hard. She hadn't met my eyes. Had she ever imagined she would be helping her own father find a care home? Her mother is chatty, comes up to help me with the check-in process when I ask what button to press next. She confirms she is here for a tour. Says the place came recommended from someone who had a relative here. She states how fussy this woman is, how many care homes she looked at before deciding on this one.

Our tour guides separate us, leading us to different parts of the home so that we might ask questions specific to our loved ones. I think uncharitably that I am competing with this other family, that we will need to make a decision quickly if we want a room here.

Double glass doors open out into the main area of the home. To the right, a group of residents are watching a black-and-white movie on television. We pass a kitchen and a public area that's being refurbished.

The room Maria shows me for Mum is being remodelled. There are plaster shards on the floor, the bed is at an angle and the armchair is in the middle of the room. It's basic, but there's a large window looking out onto a courtyard. Mum would like that.

'I'm really embarrassed to even show it to you like this.'

'It's okay. There's lovely light coming in.'

'Thanks for seeing past the works. Doing up a room after someone has left is important – your mum can put her own stamp on it.'

I wonder if the previous resident died in this room. I can't help but think how many people have died over the years in this facility. I shrug the thought away – people have to die somewhere. Still, it's a relief that no personal photo frames have been left behind. I too want Mum to make this room her own.

The memory support unit is next door to the main building. I like that the doors between the areas are kept unlocked during the day, that residents are able to move from one area to the other if they wish. It feels somehow less restraining than the highly secure dementia wing at Mum's current home.

One of the residents in the dementia wing is in the garden digging out rose bushes. Some are shuffling about on their walkers, looking for something or someone. Most are napping in their chairs or wheelchairs. Maria notes the television is off – perhaps she can turn it on? But someone expresses her disagreement loudly. Maria laughs. 'It looks like I've been told then!' She walks away, and the television remains off.

Once we've seen the facility, Maria takes me out to the courtyard, and we talk about Mum, whether it looks like this home might meet her needs. I ask the questions that have been on my mind: About how Mum might be assisted to communicate her needs given she is non-verbal. About communication with the family. About costs for the room, for extra services such as a visitation service to keep her company, flowers on her birthday.

I watch her talking, responding to each of my questions in turn – there are tiny wrinkles between her eyes and mask, her hair colour is growing out just a little, her hands move when she talks. She reminds me of my cousin Kathy, and I can't help thinking that Maria might also be hard-working, compassionate, straight shooting. It can't be easy working in aged care.

She must take many tours each week. She's selling me a room here, but she's also selling reassurance – as she talks, I'm hearing all the right things: *It's hard to put your loved one into a home. We will do our best to look after your mother. Things will not be perfect. But we will try to work with you and your family to make your mum as comfortable as possible.*

This is all I can hope for. I tell her that I'm not after perfection, or a boutique hotel for that matter. Chandeliers and fancy entryways don't interest me or Mum. I just want to know that the home is looking after Mum as well as possible so that we can enjoy the time we have left with her. My gut feeling is that we don't have long, and I want Mum to be as comfortable as possible.

As I watch Maria talk, I can feel the search for the right home finally coming to an end. I've visited more than ten homes in five months, some before Mum fell and several afterwards.

I am an hour into the tour – the longest I've had – when I declare my love for Maria. If she were a real estate agent, this is the moment where she would realise she's got me. Emotion has trumped logic, and I have Buckley's chance of being able to negotiate the daily fee for the room, or ask her to waive the 'extras' fee that Mum is not likely to get any benefit from.

But I don't care. I think I've finally found a home where I can confidently say that Mum will get decent care.

GIFT #9

Understanding

I will really listen to you

May 2023

'I don't want Mum to change care homes.'

'We've talked about this, Dennis. I don't think she's getting the care that she deserves.'

'I know. But what about the people I've met? I was sitting with John and Helen the other day, and we were talking …'

Dennis goes on to say what everyone's names are, where they are from, and divulges gossip they have shared with him. I marvel at how he might have gleaned so much, particularly as some of the narrators are unreliable – many are in various states of dementia.

'Where was Mum when you were talking with them?'

'She was in bed.'

I'm worried about Dennis. He is avoiding the care home and avoiding speaking to Mum too much when he is there. He is spending more and more time at home. Not answering the home phone. Avoiding speaking to people about Mum. Knocking back invitations from people who ask him over, who say they will drop by.

For the first time in his life, he is living alone. He's spent his whole life living in the family home with Mum and Dad.

Understanding

In the first days when Mum went into care, he said everything reminded him of her: the Greek program they watched at night, the icons which he now talks to, her empty bedroom. The nights are the hardest he says.

I too wish we weren't in this place. I wish Mum hadn't got dementia. That she hadn't had a stroke. Everything that she feared the most has happened. But there is no choice but to deal with it, just as she is dealing with it. But I don't have to go home to an empty house at night.

'I'm sad too, Dennis. But we've got to do what's best for Mum. And right now, I think she needs to be somewhere where she has her own room, some peace and quiet, and decent care. She's been good to everyone all her life. She deserves that.'

'Still, I'll miss the people there …'

I pause, think carefully about asking the next question.

'Is it easier to be with the other residents there than it is to be with Mum?'

He readily agrees and his eyes pool. 'I wish she had just gone in her sleep. I don't want her to be tortured like this.'

I wish it too, even though I don't think I'll ever be ready for Mum to die.

'Mum seems reasonably comfortable. Content even. And I know for a fact that you will get used to the new place. You will connect with people there too.'

Dennis acknowledges that that will likely happen. He has a trusting face, is a great listener. Older people and children gravitate to him. He has an almost child-like demeanour. I know he will be fine.

I'd discussed the new home with Dennis. We'd looked at it online and had arranged a visit together. He'd found things to fault: 'The doors are too narrow. There's no parking. And there are no paths on the footpath outside to take Mum for a walk.'

'Dennis, you will get used to it, I know you will.'

After so many visits to care homes, I've finally found one where I believe Mum will get good care. We decide to sleep on it, and I can get in touch to secure our place after the weekend.

I don't think Dennis's reservations are about the home. He hates change, is struggling with so many losses, one after the other. I feel guilty that Dennis is spending so much time alone at home. I ring him daily, try and see him at least once a week, and am trying my best to accommodate his needs as well as Mum's. Our cousin Jorge drops by to help with gardening and to finish the painting, and also rings often. My cousins Kathy, Dim and Georgia ring regularly. The neighbour drops by with food. Dennis talks with people on the street on his daily walks. But still, there's no getting away from the fact that Mum is declining. And we can't do anything to stop it.

*

'Are you sure Chrisoula's been accepted? She has very high needs you know …'

Understanding

The client services manager lets the sentence hang, suggesting that it's going to be hard for Mum to find a care place. But I don't need to be told how high her needs are: I can see that for myself.

I'm here to give the mandatory two weeks' notice that Mum is leaving the home where she currently resides. According to the contract, it's all that's required.

'Yes, I'm very sure,' I say. I've been careful to get Mum's new care place accepted in writing.

'As a matter of fact, a single room has just become available. But I'm needing an answer by tomorrow, as there's someone waiting for it ...'

I wonder how a room has become available so suddenly. I wonder if they are going to kick someone out of their room in order to accommodate Mum in a bid not to lose a paying customer. I recognise the sales tactic of subtly pressuring us to decide quickly, but I'm not falling for it as I did when we first came here. I dislike this new cynical, slightly bitter side to myself. I'm not as trusting as I was a few months ago.

'Thank you, but we are good. Just let me know if there is anything else I need to do.'

I make sure to follow up with an email confirming our discussion, copy the clinical services manager in with details of the new place for a handover. I don't want to leave anything to chance.

*

I'm waiting inside the new care home for an initial meeting to talk about Mum's care, but Dennis isn't here. He's usually early. Soon, I see him outside the door. He looks like he's been crying, like he's about to blow up.

'Are you okay, Dennis?'

'No, I'm not okay. I'm sick of this. If this place doesn't work out, I'm just going to pick Mum up and take her home. I can't do this anymore. I don't want any more changes.'

His hands are shaking as he tries to manage the RAT test. His face is red, and his voice is getting louder.

I think about how he will be during the meeting, who is listening to us in the nearby offices. I keep my voice calm and low.

'Alright. You don't have to be here right now. Do you want to walk around for a bit, and then come back after the meeting? We can set Mum's room up together.'

'No, I've been walking around for ages. I need to do this. Let's just get it over and done with. There's a big nursing home on the hill. Maybe we should send Mum there.' His eyes dart towards the horizon. He is close to tears.

'Dennis, we've just come from a big place. And we agreed on this place last week. What are you talking about?' Though I'm trying to be calm, I can hear my own voice rising. I need to calm down.

I tell him that the meeting is probably not a great time to cry. He says, 'I will cry if I want to …'

Understanding

The intake worker is professional, warm. She spends almost two hours asking about Mum – what she eats, how she sleeps, what her preferences are, and relevant medical issues. She acknowledges how hard it is for family members, and that over time we can develop trust in the home to look after Mum so we can go back to enjoying time with her. She tells us the best place to park; where the paths are around the home to go for a walk with a wheelchair; and how to operate the television so we can find some Greek content for Mum. The meeting focuses exclusively on Mum's needs. It is yet another reassuring sign that we have made the right decision to move her. I compare this to the short pre-admission meeting at the other facility, where I felt largely talked at. Already, I feel more comfortable here.

Dennis is quiet. He sits by the window. Nods.

We set Mum's room up. Put pictures against the window, a pot plant on her side table, neatly fold her clothes, place perfume on her vanity. We try to make it homely.

As soon as we walk out, Dennis's face reddens again, tears threaten.

'How do you think that went?' I say tentatively.

'It's good to know there is more parking on the grounds. And that there is a back path leading to the shops. Still, there aren't as many Greeks here.'

'Dennis, I know this is hard, but already I feel that Mum will be in better hands here after just a few meetings than I did with the other aged care home over two months. We are doing this for Mum. Now, you can't go home in this state. Let's go for a coffee. We'll talk it over.'

'I don't want to talk. I'm sick of talking. I just want to go home.'

'Dennis, I'm really worried about you. You seem to be crying more and more. Seem more upset, more often. It's natural to be sad and stressed at this time. I feel that too. But we need to try to do the things that keep us well so that we can function.'

Every suggestion family and friends have made to Dennis these past few weeks about how he might cope with the changes seems to have fallen on deaf ears. It's like we're having the same conversations over and over. I feel like I've been carrying Mum and Dennis for so long. I'm exhausted and overwhelmed. I can't keep doing this.

'I'm sorry, Dennis, but I can't help you and Mum at the same time. I can't help you if you don't help yourself. I can be your sister, I can even be your friend. But I can't be your mother or your psychologist. You've got to get help.'

By now, we've walked the block several times. The light is going and the only shop that's open in the strip is the bottle shop. It's time to go home.

Dennis's shoulders are slumped. I wonder if I've gone too far, been too harsh. But I'm at my wits' end.

He looks at me, nods. 'I'll ring my doctor tomorrow.'

*

Understanding

At the entry to Mum's current aged care home, there's been a sign on the door for a few weeks, stating that visitors need to do a RAT test, wear a mask and sanitise their hands because there have been cases of Covid in the facility. Now, there's a new sign on the door: *Do not enter*. There's been regular updates on the app, which I often forget to check.

I'm taken aback, even though I already know Covid cases have appeared in Mum's ward. For the past few weeks, they have been confined to the memory support area downstairs. I rang earlier this afternoon to check if I could still visit Mum. I was told there are now nine cases on her ward, up from six a few days back. I hesitate before asking: *Does Mum have it? No, she doesn't*.

There are four days to go before she moves into a new care home. Please don't let her get Covid now.

I take a breath as I press the buzzer to be let in. I'm ready to argue my case about why I should be able to see Mum. But the man who opens the door takes only a cursory glance at the single line on the RAT test, waves me towards the monitor that takes my temperature and details of who I'm visiting.

There are several women sitting in the plush armchairs under the oversized chandelier that graces the reception area. When I first visited the home, I'd thought they were waiting for their families, but I now know it's just where they like to congregate. They look out onto the almost empty car park. Everything seems normal.

I make my way down the corridor towards Mum's wing, but two imposing floor-to-ceiling white doors bar the area. They're plastered with an ominous warning in red letters: *RED ZONE: COVID-19 AFFECTED ZONE. PLEASE DO NOT ENTER.*

I try the door, expecting it to be locked, but it swings open. I tap in the code to Mum's wing and round the corner. The nurses' station is unoccupied. There are no staff in the corridors either, most of the residents' doors closed. The evidence of what is happening here is everywhere: yellow waste bins run the length of the hall; trolleys outside several rooms are laden with blue gowns, gloves, masks and pump packs of sanitiser; air purifiers are whirring. I'm already kitted up with a mask and face shield but wonder if I should gown up too. I walk the perimeter of the unit and find a few staff in the common area getting dinner trays ready. They look surprised to see me.

'I'm here to see Mum. Should I gown up too?' I ask sheepishly. Surely that won't be necessary.

'Yes, it's probably best. You don't want to risk catching it, giving it to others.'

I don the mask, but don't put on gloves. That feels like it's going too far. I don't know whether to laugh or cry with the absurdity of it all. *Four days to go.*

In her room, Mum looks up at me from her low bed. She is pleased and befuddled. Asks the same questions she usually does. *Where did you come from? How did you get here? Where are you?* Though some of her questions don't make sense, I go

Understanding

through the standard phrases in a bid to give her a sense of time and place, to hit on something that will make her face relax into understanding. *I came from home. I came in my car. It's Sunday. It's nearly dinner time.* I lower my mask so she can see my lips, my face.

Her roommate dozes in her wheelchair next door, her TV on in the background. Mum's television is off, and I wonder what she has been doing all day. But she looks rested, calm. I tell myself again that's what matters. When it's explained to her why everyone needs to stay in their rooms, she nods, her words undecipherable. She doesn't seem particularly perturbed.

I've brought fried sardines, home-made bread and grapes – all things she loves. I explain that George made the bread, and that he is visiting his dad in the care home at this moment. They too have several cases of Covid. My father-in-law is going stir crazy cooped up in his room. There is a sympathetic look on her face. *Poor thing.*

She ignores the fish, but picks at the grapes, distracted by the television which is now switched on. I go around the room, packing clothes and toiletries she is unlikely to need over coming days so that there is less to take on her last day. When she asks what I'm doing, I remind her that in four days she will be moving to a new care home. She sounds surprised. I explain again that there she will have her own room. That a Greek priest visits once a month. That there are other Greek speakers living there. I'm not sure if I'm trying to reassure myself, or her. I hope

I've made the right decision. After nearly two months here, Mum seems settled. And now I'm going to uproot her.

'What about home?' She looks at me, testing. Will I give the right answer this time?

'We can visit home if you like. But you know you can't live there anymore. It's too hard …' I hold my breath. How will she respond this time?

She swears crudely. I clearly didn't give her the answer she wanted. But the words are delivered with humour and impeccable comedic timing, a cheeky gleam in her eyes. We both laugh.

Mum's roommate stirs. I greet her, trepidatious, waiting to see what mood she will be in, whether she will start screaming or complaining. She asks me to *please* switch on her light in a sugary tone. And could I *please* move the curtain aside that is blocking her view into Mum's space. I consider denying her the second request but figure it's hard being wheelchair- and room-bound. Her being able to see us isn't such a big imposition. I do as she says, wait for her to take it further, but she doesn't. Mum looks at me. She doesn't need to use words – her eyes say it all. *What does she want now? Is she behaving herself?*

Food is delivered to the room by two masked and gowned carers. They are familiar. Even after eight weeks, I have only learnt a handful of names. Still, I've gotten to recognise those who have kind eyes, who will volunteer a little snippet about how Mum's day has gone. Mum is unfailingly polite to everyone,

Understanding

showers them with compliments in her jumbled Greek. To me they admit they don't understand a word she says, but she is *so cute*. They call her 'Mamma' and her face lights up, her hands reach out to stroke them, keep them close. She needs them to pay her attention, to look after her. Even now, she knows that it's best to be kind, that people are more likely to help you. I'm proud of her: she has no words, and yet she's still holding her own. I too want to implore the carers: *Please look after my beautiful mother because we no longer can.*

As I spoon food into Mum's mouth, I'm reminded of feeding my children when they were infants. *Mouth opening and closing. Chest raising and falling. Life waxing and waning.* I think again about how what begins must end – a circle that goes around and around. I am glad to be here with Mum, to be helping her in her time of greatest need.

Midway through the meal, Mum sneezes several times. A splatter of mash and beans sprays onto my hands and face before I can pull the spoon away. I regret not donning gloves, wash my hands carefully after the meal. I can't afford to get Covid, mostly because I won't be able to visit Mum. And if George becomes a close contact, he won't be able to visit his parents.

Mum's roommate starts complaining loudly to a carer who comes in to take her tray. *The mash is cold. Nurse, what is this? I don't like this. Please listen to me. Can you heat the food up again?* The carer takes the plate dutifully away. I think about the hourly rate she must be getting. I'm betting it's nowhere nearly enough for her to sweat into her PPE and deal with the likes of Mum's roommate.

The nurse on the afternoon shift stands at the door, mixing Mum's medications into a cup. She is one person I have gotten to know reasonably well, a no-nonsense older woman, her chest buxom in her shirt, her face lined. She competently takes charge of the common area each night as she goes around dispensing drugs and instructions: *Betty's chair needs adjusting. Maria needs help eating. Come on Anastasia, you can eat more than that!* She exudes confidence and humanity. I know that her elderly mother lives overseas. She and her siblings can check in on her through cameras set up in the house and yard. She has told me the needs of most elderly are surprisingly simple to meet. She's good at making people comfortable.

Tonight, she is agitated and stands outside the door mixing Mum's drugs more rigorously than usual. All it takes is a few sympathetic words from me and she's off.

'I'm sick of Covid, and all this ...' Her arm sweeps across the corridor behind her. 'It's hard to get four anti-viral tablets into them in one pop, poor things. They are all stuck in their rooms, and most don't understand why. People can't visit. They're not eating. I hate coming to work when things get to this.'

I tell her that it must be so hard to come to this point again after what they went through over the lockdowns. She nods, gives Mum her medicine, and moves down the corridor.

Understanding

I prepare myself for the ritual of saying goodbye to Mum: pack up the food I have bought, lower her bed to the ground and put mats in place on either side of the bed in case she rolls out. Usually, I give her a kiss through my mask, but tonight I don't dare.

On the way out, I bin my mask, shield and gown. Stepping out into the cold night air is a relief. I swipe at the sweat that has pooled under my eyes, think of the carers who have a long shift ahead of them. It will be hours yet before they can go home to their own families.

*

The day has come for Mum to be discharged. Dennis has driven to the home, is waiting outside so that he doesn't have to do a RAT test, don full PPE.

In the corridor, I pull on the gear and round the corner. I report to the nurse dispensing drugs, tell him that Mum is being discharged today, that I need to pick up her medications. And is there anything else we need to do?

He looks confused. *There was nothing in the discharge meeting this morning ...*

'Oh. Can I speak with the clinical manager?'

He goes to ask one of the personal carers where she might be. 'She's working downstairs.'

Someone else overhears, says she will be in at 10.

'I can't wait that long. I've got a taxi booked. We have to leave this morning.'

He'll get the nurse.

I gown up and go to Mum's room. She is sitting in her wheelchair. Her roommate naps in her wheelchair next to her.

The charge nurse finally arrives, someone I've never seen before. She stands in the hallway so she doesn't have to gown up.

'We're being discharged today. I told the client services officer and the clinical manager. But no one seems to know anything about it.'

'You will need to advise the new provider that there is a Covid outbreak in the facility.'

'I didn't know this was up to me. I thought they would have been told in a handover …'

'No, it's your responsibility. We can't let her go. You will have to tell them and see what they say.'

I turn away, don't trust myself to speak or contain my rising anger.

My mind reels. If I declare that there is Covid in Mum's ward, Mum will not be allowed to go. She tested negative on PCR and RAT tests just a day ago. What sort of risk does she pose? It feels as if we will never get out of here.

It's only then that I notice the big round red dot on the door to the room.

'Does someone in this room have Covid?' I ask, incredulous.

Understanding

She nods.

'Is that person my mother?' I can hear the fear, the anger in my voice. Could it be that she has Covid, that no one has told me? I wouldn't be surprised, I think bitterly.

'No.'

'Okay, so the other person has Covid?' I look back at her roommate. The curtain is pulled back between the two spaces. There are no masks, no air purifiers in the room. Her roommate leans towards Mum's table, takes a magazine from it.

There's a small nod from the nurse. I ask why I wasn't told, and she mumbles something about privacy, about it only coming back positive last night.

'Do you want to speak to the executive director?'

'Yes, yes I do.'

I can tell she is relieved. Someone who is paid better than her can deal with it. With *me*.

I pace the room like a caged lion. I am furious. The nurse comes back, tells me she has conveyed the message to the ED. I ring the other provider. There is no option now. Mum is in the same room with someone who has tested positive with Covid. Putting the residents of another home into a risky, potential lockdown situation is unthinkable.

The clinical manager at the other facility is sympathetic. As Mum is a close contact, she will need to have another PCR test. If the result is negative, she will be accepted, though once at the new home, she will need to isolate for three days and have RAT tests for seven days. I cancel the taxi. Text my brother about the new developments. Pace some more, and, after half an hour, realise that the ED isn't going to come. It's nearly 11 now. Mum looks at me, concerned. Her eyes question me: *What's going on?*

Mum is so vulnerable in her bed, but still able to intuit my anger and distress, and it makes me pause. I think about how Mum has always shown me that you need to step into the shoes of others, try to empathise with how it is for them – and in doing so, more often than not, you can find common ground. It's a skill that was formally taught in my social work training, and it's one that I've honed in my professional practice. Mum's example has helped me foster connections with people, helped me engage meaningfully with them when they are angry or upset. I need to be patient to navigate this next challenge in order to protect Mum's best interests. I need to put my anger to one side to think more clearly.

I tell her I'm trying to work things out, apologise for being stressed. I encourage her to try and get some rest.

I ring the reception area, leave a message for the ED. I'm told she's in a meeting. I realise nothing is going to happen unless I act decisively. I tell the receptionist I will wait outside her office. There, I can hear the ED speaking on the phone to someone – it sounds like she is trying to placate someone else who is complaining.

She comes to the corridor, looks wary.

Understanding

I tell her that Mum was to be discharged today, explain the morning's events. I say the new provider is insisting on a PCR test. She says she is happy to organise that. Will Mum be assured of a bed until she moves? *Yes.* Is a single room available until we leave. *No.*

She says she is sorry the message did not get passed on about Mum's discharge. *There are lots of agency staff. What with the lockdowns and all …* She will look into how that happened … I tell her how disappointed I am. She acknowledges my concerns, but there's no sense she's going to lose any sleep over it.

I go back to Mum; tell her she will be moving in a few days, and that I'll be back tomorrow. There's the push and pull. *Where am I going? Why am I going?*

Once I've placated her, I discard my PPE in the hallway, meet Dennis in the front. He's confused and upset. We walk around the block several times, both of us venting our frustration. We agree it's poor. When he leaves, I ring George and offload some more. Finally, I march around the block, venting to Kathy.

I go home and write a very terse email to the CEO confirming what we spoke about and reiterating my disappointment about the train of events. I read it over several times. It's assertive, clear, if a bit long. I press the 'send' button.

*

The clinical manager comes in, hands me the negative PCR result. Apologises that she wasn't here yesterday, but she was on annual leave. Doesn't know how the message wasn't conveyed. She is back in charge now, asks if I need anything else. I reiterate how disappointed I am. She too acknowledges this, thinks the breakdown in communication was due to agency staff. She says that the customer service office will address my queries about Covid. I thank her. I wonder if I hadn't sent the terse email, whether she would have come down to speak with me. I realised I'm being managed. A potentially dissatisfied customer.

The next day, I see that the last of Mum's clothes have been put into a pile in the wardrobe, that there is nothing else to take. Mum is showered and ready to go. Personal carers come into the room. One of the more gregarious ones, the one who always imparted a few snippets of information about Mum – *she ate a good breakfast, she had a shower today* – gives her a hug.

'It's sad. The best ones always leave,' he says.

Another talks about how good she is, how gentle. She makes it easy to care for her.

But then her roommate starts calling at the top of her voice, 'Nurse, nurse, I need to go to the toilet!' The carers turn reluctantly, go back to work.

As we leave, I can hear Mum's roommate calling out in the bathroom, see a dirty continence aid on her bed between the gap in the curtains. There won't be any teary goodbyes. Once again, I won't be sorry to see the back of this room.

Understanding

As I am taking off my PPE in the no-man's land between the locked-down and open wards, the customer service officer flies through the double doors of the corridor. She says Mum is so *cute*. And as we've been paying on a month-by-month basis a month in advance, any unused funds will be reimbursed.

Both she and the clinical manager stand at the door to see us out. I thank them for their care, for responding to queries quickly. Always my mother's daughter – find *something positive to say*. They tell me that if there is anything that the new provider needs, they are always available. We stand awkwardly, and I think they are just as relieved as I am when the taxi arrives.

We go out the door and don't look back.

*

Mum was a bit confused on coming to the new home, but as always, didn't complain. I've been staying with her during the day while she's in isolation, offering reassurance and what I hope is a grounding presence every time she wakes.

The workers need to kit up every time they come in, and they've largely left us alone except to bring in food, and to change and turn Mum. I stand in the doorway of the toilet while they change Mum. So far, no one has given me cause for concern. The room is large enough that the hoist can be manoeuvred around the bed, that the two workers needed to shift Mum can stand comfortably around her. I'm glad for the cocoon-like feeling of the room, that the bed is well away from busyness of the corridor, and that the window offers a vantage point to the outside. An endearing older man offers me sandwiches, tea, which makes me feel nurtured too.

It's our third day in, and Mum naps. I've holed up in the armchair next to the bed, the television on silent. I've set the room up with a few pot plants, some icons, and several photos, which are placed on the walls and along the windowsills: portraits of our children with Mum and Dennis, one of Dim and her kids and grandkids; one of Mum and her sister at her granddaughter Sophia's wedding. I think back to just a year ago, when Mum danced with Sophia at her wedding. The sisters wore matching red and blue sparkling tops. It feels like a lifetime ago. When Mum is awake, I use the pictures to prompt conversation, tell her what everyone is doing, how they are looking forward to visit once they are allowed. Mum nods, and there are little looks of recognition. But mostly she naps.

With all this time on my hands, I can't help but reflect on the past few years that have led us here: the lockdowns, Mum's diagnosis, the many challenges George's parents have had, and the significant impact on our family. Over the last year alone, there's been Mum's sudden decline, her fall at home and in hospital, the transition to care, and now the move to a new home. It's been a lot.

I'm drawn away from my grim musings by the view from the window. A few carers are having their lunch in the autumn

Understanding

sun. A resident approaches them. They chat briefly. On finishing her lunch, one of the carers joins the resident on the garden bench, chatting companionably before going back inside. The resident places the hat over his eyes and snoozes in the sunshine.

The image is deeply reassuring. Though I couldn't have imagined Mum being in this position even a year ago, my confidence she will be comfortable and safe here grows each day.

Now that she is in good hands, we can just try to make the most of whatever time we have left with her.

*

'You know you could have asked to see it?' says the nurse.

We're talking about a pressure sore on Mum's bottom. It's another legacy of the previous home.

She gives me an even look, as if it's bleedingly obvious.

'Do you want to see it now?'

I don't want to. But I need to. 'Yes, of course.'

She pulls out her phone, finds the image. The close-up of the pressure sore looks like a bruise, it's edges dark, the surrounding skin pink and inflamed. I fight back nausea and guilt. Not only does this wound look painful, it's in the most intimate of places on my mother's body.

The nurse tells me they'll need to get a doctor to look at it. It will need to be medicated and cleaned daily. To prevent further damage, Mum will likely be kept off her bottom and turned regularly to avoid it flaring up again. She won't be able to spend much time in her wheelchair in the common area.

You could have asked to see it. In the weeks before we left the previous home, Mum had developed a pressure sore. The worker stated that they were treating it, but nothing more was said. On the occasions that I asked the nurse about it, there were brief responses. *Yes, it's healing. It's all good. It's under control.*

It appears it wasn't under control. Though I feel a little berated by the nurse's terse manner, it's clear we are in a place where there is more open communication, and it seems to me, more appropriate action when things go wrong. It's the best we can hope for. I take hold of Mum's hand. Give it a squeeze. She smiles, looks bewildered. *My poor, poor mother.*

*

I'd been dreading filling out yet again the slew of forms relating to taking residence in an aged care home: a charter of resident rights, a privacy statement, a leisure and lifestyle document, a contract numbering over 60 pages. Thankfully, they settle Mum in first, then the forms are drip fed to me.

At the previous home, there was a hefty form where I'd stated what Mum's leisure and lifestyle preferences were. I felt more and more cynical as I made my way through each page; felt increasingly doubtful that someone would even read it, much less action some of the statements made. I don't recall any

Understanding

questions where I could state that Mum wasn't literate, numerate or able to communicate effectively verbally. She wouldn't be able to participate in many activities, except as an observer.

I'm glad that the equivalent form at this care home is only two pages long. It asks simple, relevant questions. I imagine it will actually be read, that someone should be able to take something from it to make Mum's life a little bit more comfortable here. I fill it out while Mum naps: she has four siblings; she came to Australia in 1965; she likes the garden; enjoys being massaged; she would like Greek liturgy playing on her death bed, surrounded by family. I can only guess at some of these things. Perhaps I am projecting. Still, I make the statements in firm block letters.

There is a form called an advanced care directive. A nurse had explained it at length during the pre-admission meeting. She'd said it was important that Mum's preferences are stated clearly. Do we want her to stay at the care home if she is nearing end of life, or would we like her to be managed in hospital? What if she stops breathing – do we consent to resuscitation? What about a breathing machine? I'd filled in such a form at the previous home – I barely remember what I wrote. They were keen that I do it quickly, in case anything happened to Mum.

With support from staff, I state what is important – Mum only having procedures that lead to better quality of life, receiving end-of-life care in the care home if possible, not being revived should she lose consciousness. I'd checked in with Dennis, who'd agreed: our main concern now is Mum's comfort.

I'm typing up the form at my desk when George comes in, asks what I'm doing.

'I'm filling in this advanced care directive. Did you do one of these for your Dad? It says a doctor needs to sign it.'

He vaguely remembers doing one, can't remember who signed it.

'There is so much that doesn't relate to Mum because she's lost so much capacity already …'

George puts his hands on my shoulders. I burst into tears.

*

We're a few weeks into Mum's stay at the new aged care home. When I come in, the nurse reports that Mum's pressure sore is better, she is getting up every few days, that she is eating a little. I feel reassured: they are monitoring her food intake, seem to be keeping an eye on her pain and discomfort.

Every time I come in, I ask a lot of questions. I'm still reeling from the previous home; feel the need to be hypervigilant. I talk with the woman who inducted Mum into the home, ask her whether I am being a nuisance. She reassures me that my questions are valid. She says that the family members who are the most problematic are those that come in with very high expectations about what is possible, who have trouble understanding that this is not a one-on-one environment where a worker can be with your loved one exclusively. She goes on to say that it can also be challenging when families, who are so often having trouble dealing with their own lack of control and grief over their loved one's trajectory, lash out at workers. I assure her I'm not one to lash out. I have inherited my mother's politeness gene.

I make my way to Mum's room, and her face is a mixture of confusion and joy on seeing me – thankfully more joy than confusion. Dennis and I fear the day when she might not recognise us at all.

I put up her bed, give her a kiss.

'How are you, Mamma?'

'Last night I nearly died,' she says. It's rare these days for her to say a complete sentence that makes sense.

'Why do you say that, Mamma?'

She mumbles something about the night. I don't understand, ask several more questions, but get nowhere.

'Mum, we're in a new place. You have a sore on your bottom. I know it's not comfortable. But you are not going to die anytime soon I don't think.' I try to smile reassuringly. My jaunty tone is irritating, even to me.

She nods, her attention deflecting to young people on the television. She mentions something about Sofia, her sister, looks out the window to the workmen in the courtyard, wonders who they are.

Mum and I have talked about death a lot. There is some comfort in knowing that she is ready, that she has made peace with the idea of dying.

I'm not ready. I cling to her, selfishly. *Just a little more time please, just a little more time.* Even though Mum is now so incapacitated she can't walk, eat by herself, communicate clearly or toilet herself, moaning in pain every time carers turn her, I still don't want her to go.

That night I dream I'm in a cubicle with my cousin Dim. She is upset about something, can barely hold back tears. There is a huge space behind us that feels like a stadium. Through a door I can see people and an ambulance. Someone is administering CPR, and I know instantly it's Mum on the receiving end. I run to her as fast as I can, screaming, expecting her to be dead, but she is lying there, nude, breathing calmly. I cradle her in my lap, and she fits there like a baby. Soon, she stands up, white flesh gleaming in the moonlight. I'm surprised she can walk, follow her across the grass and into a pool. We swim together. Soon, I am looking down on her and see another version of Mum, who is a few metres away, and she is dying. I am paralysed and confused, can't do anything about it, and don't know which Mum to turn to …

I wake, feeling unsettled. Emmanuel is walking around the house, getting ready for work. The heater pumps warm air into the cold winter morning. I try to get back to sleep, but it eludes me yet again.

Understanding

*

'*Tha pethano.*' I'm going to die.

I open my mouth to tell Mum she's not dying, but quickly re-think my words. We're sitting outside in the winter sunshine, in a courtyard garden with raised beds planted with young carrots and parsley. She struggles to open her eyes.

'*Ti niotheis?*' What are you feeling?

She is unable to say. Did she sleep last night? She nods: *Yes*. Is she in pain? *No*. She looks so vacant. I wonder if she is finally succumbing to despair. I feel pangs of guilt, think perhaps I should have come in yesterday. But the almost daily visits are taking their toll, and home fires need to be stoked. I need to protect my own health to keep going. Over a year has passed since Mum needed advanced care. I'd seen her every second day since then: there were times I'd seen her every day.

When I'd arrived this morning, Mum was being sponged down. There were three carers, and a hoist, packed into the room. I was asked to wait in the hallway. I gathered that she'd just opened her bowels, and the bandage covering her pressure sore had become soiled. A nurse was called in to change it. I could hear Mum moaning in discomfort through the closed door. I'd held my breath, felt queasy – it's so hard to hear her pain. A carer had wheeled her out. I'd asked that she sit up for a while, get out of bed while I'm here. I thought it might do her good to be in the sun, perhaps have lunch in the dining room.

I wonder now whether I am doing more harm than good and take her back inside, where lunch is being served. A Greek-speaking resident calls us over, checks to see if there is room to seat Mum. When we've wedged Mum's wheelchair nearby, she hobbles over. Says it's good to see Mum up. That she herself went to the local church today for a 40-day commemorative service for a former resident. *He was a lovely man …* Her voice trails off.

I wonder if the man that died had resided in Mum's room. It must be hard for the residents when someone dies, when the deceased's room is occupied by someone else.

'It's great that you can still go. Mum used to go regularly,' I say.

'I go while I can. Who knows how long it will last …' she says.

'Mum, we can go with a taxi if you want …'

Her look says, *perhaps*. The logistics of organising an accessible taxi, manoeuvring her heavy wheelchair into the crowded church, and then organising a return taxi, feels onerous, particularly if she is feeling like she is today.

The resident hobbles over to her seat, asks one of the carers for a bib for the woman sitting beside her. It's reassuring that some residents look after each other, despite their own problems. I'm pleased that there are a handful of Greek speakers here so that Mum can at least hear her first language.

Mum barely opens her mouth to eat a few spoonfuls of food, and it's clear I should stop trying. We return to her room.

Understanding

She naps in her chair while I potter around: re-folding clothes, placing perfume, a foot scrub, and a body lotion that Dim and Kathy have brought over on the weekend into the bathroom cabinet; setting up a laundry bag in her wardrobe for carers to place dirty woollens for me to take home. These little rituals make me feel as if I'm doing something useful, even though they will likely make little difference to Mum. I'm trying to put our stamp on this room, create a little piece of home for her. I finally sit down, stare out the window, half an eye on the movie playing silently in the background.

When Mum wakes, I tell her in jaunty tones that it's time for a manicure, try to get her to put her hands in a bowl of soapy water, but they keep dropping away. I soon give up, just clip her nails and file down the thick stubborn one that the clipper can't get around, even though I know that the carers will do this at some point. Her hands are pale and smooth. I realise that probably for the first time in her life, her hands aren't working. They have worked so hard, so constantly since she was a little girl: gardening, cooking, cleaning. They have sewn thousands upon thousands of nighties. When my children were small, she helped look after them, cooked us meals, helped clean our house. I can't help but think that no matter what I offer her now, it will never be enough.

I think of all this work as I massage Mum's hands, careful to be gentle with her little finger, which is permanently bent. Its stiffness horrified me when I was younger. I would try to straighten it back, but it wouldn't budge. It's a grim reminder of a freak accident when she was a young mum in her thirties, new to Australia. As a child, I never tired of hearing the story of how it happened. Mum patiently narrated it every time I asked.

'I had just finished sewing a batch of nighties, and I needed to get the boss to take them away, and to order more work. We didn't have a phone then. I had to walk to the payphone at the milkbar. I left you and your brother sitting in front of the television. Dennis wasn't yet at school; you were a toddler. I told Dennis not to open the door to anyone. You begged and begged to come with me, but I said, "No". I wanted to get home quickly.

'I rushed to the milk bar, and on the way back, a car rammed an ambulance, which mounted the footpath. I was run over. On hearing the commotion, the neighbours came rushing out. I don't remember anything, but apparently, I'd called out, "My children, my children ..."'

At this point in the story, Mum would look at me with her astute blue eyes, as if to say, *See how mothers, even those who are nearly dead, always look out for their children first!*

'Yiayia Yiannoula from across the road, God bless her soul, ran to see if you were okay. The door was locked. Dennis wouldn't let her in!'

The story of Mum's bent finger has been passed down to Dolores and Emmanuel. They too are intrigued by their yiayia's bent finger.

Understanding

I tell them that their yiayia was on the news that night. That she was lucky to be alive. Along with her finger, she broke her hip and numerous ribs, lost hearing in one ear. She was in hospital for months. It would be two years before she was well enough to work again. Uncle Dennis and I had to stay with Yiayia's sister Sofia, who had my cousins Kathy and Georgia at the time, was pregnant with Dim …'

When I tell the story, I add my own little embellishments: Had I gone with their yiayia that day, as a toddler, likely I wouldn't be here now. And nor would they.

After the massage, I pull down the photo of our family on Mum's wall. I tell her what Emmanuel is up to, that he is enjoying his apprenticeship. I tell her about Dolores, who is on an extended trip overseas, show her photos. I suggest we should try and ring her when the times align. She smiles, and a look of warmth comes over her face.

I put the photo back. Mum looks dozy. I'm relieved when a carer comes in to put her back to bed. She's been sitting on her bottom for more than two hours. My attempts at getting her out don't feel as if they've given her, or me, much joy.

That night, I dream that my brother and I have taken Mum out for a walk in her wheelchair. She is emaciated, all bones and sagging skin, barely able to sit up. I return her to the care home scooped up in my arms. She morphs into a baby swaddled in a sheet. I wrap my arms around her protectively, wondering how it is that my once-solidly built mother has become so small.

GIFT #10

Kindness

I will speak kind words

September 2023

Spring has taken hold in our garden: bees are buzzing across lush lavender bushes, the fruit trees are budding, and a luxurious bed of silverbeet is regenerating faster than we can possibly eat it or give it away. There is the pleasant feel of sunshine on bare skin, the promise of warmer days ahead.

Despite all this light and regeneration, my spirit feels dark. Mum has lost 12 kilos in the last month. The staff are alarmed – they had noticed she was losing weight, but it wasn't until her monthly weigh in that they realised just how much. Over the next week, there's a flurry of activity: they get the doctor in, the dietitian; take blood tests, monitor her food intake. No matter what I bring her to eat, she refuses to take more than a few mouthfuls. Her meals are taken back to the kitchen, almost untouched. Mum, who has always had such a healthy appetite, and who has spent her whole life feeding others, no longer wants to eat. It feels like the final blow.

Before visiting Mum later that afternoon, I walk with my friend Sarah-Jane, whose father also has dementia. Sarah-Jane works in a funeral home, is a funeral celebrant. I feel comfortable talking with her about my concerns, am grateful to get another perspective on what Mum is going through. I babble, confused and upset. Sarah-Jane lets me cry, listens patiently while I talk about not being able to make things better for Mum. She talks gently about Mum's right to dignity, alludes to the fact that Mum is probably getting ready to pass. Sarah-Jane talks about the need for me to care for myself. To take a breath and reset after yet another downward step in Mum's trajectory. I'm grateful for her kindness, hope that I have listened as generously as she has on the occasions when she shared her own challenges in the past.

I cry again when I get home, tell George I've been filling my days with activity as a way of coping.

I cry again when my cousin Kathy rings me on the way to Mum's.

I can't help Mum. I can't make this better. I can't control this. I find it hard to know what to do to help. This is a shitty disease.

We rant and cry together.

Her father is also showing signs of dementia. He's been recently admitted to a residential care home. She's visiting several times a week, is often taking calls from the home about managing his care. Kathy says *she* is all over the place. That she went shopping this morning, bought some eggplants, but couldn't find them when she got home. Doesn't even know if she paid for them. They cost a fortune too! We laugh through the tears.

She agrees it's not fair what is happening, that a beautiful person like her *Theia* Chrisoula doesn't deserve it. That no one deserves it.

I feel spent after all this crying, but lighter. I drop into a fresh produce barn on the way to Mum. Buy her custard, biscuits that will be easy to chew. And some eggplants for Kathy, which I will drop off on my way home. They might make her laugh.

When I get to the care home, Mum seems more alert. I feed her the custard. Massage her face. Ring my brother so she can hear his voice. Notice that her colour is better today. I feel the familiar push and pull. I'm not ready for her to go, but this is not a way to live. I think about turning the television on to distract her, but she doesn't seem to get any joy out of that. She used to watch Greek shows with Dennis each night, but she got to a point where she didn't understand the dialogue, and it distressed her. Along with long telephone calls with her sisters, and walks around the block, these things fell to the wayside one by one in the months before her fall.

She sleeps and wakes. Sees me by her side, looks reassured that I am still here. I tell her I love her.

'*Siga!*' No kidding. We laugh.

My distress from earlier this morning morphs into love and gratefulness. No matter what happens, it will be okay.

*

'*Eimai etoimi.*' I'm ready.

'Ready for what?'

'*To taxithi.*' The trip.

Mum's laying flat in the bed, her eyes a faded watery blue. The corners of her eyes are wet. Is she crying?

'What trip, Mum?'

She tries but she can't get her tongue around the words, and they slip away. She goes back to staring at the ceiling. After a while, I tell her I might leave to give her a chance to rest, but she says, '*Oxi.*' No.

I turn the television on, set it to mute. When Mum closes her eyes, I check work emails, respond to a message on the family chat. It's now 5 pm. I've come from work, haven't been home since 7 this morning – wonder if there are enough leftovers from last night for dinner.

A carer places a tray of food next to the food I've brought in. I hold Mum's hand as she naps, wakes, murmurs. The food gets cold. It gets taken away. When Mum wakes again, I ask if she needs anything: *A sip of water? Is she comfortable?* Tuck her in, straighten her blanket. I feel the urge to get in with her, hold her.

'I should head home, Mamma.'

This time, she doesn't fight it, lets me give her a kiss.

*

When I next visit Mum, her mouth is open to a dark 'O', her chest seems not to be moving. I stand there a few minutes, hold my breath, walk around the bed to take a better look. The up and down movements are small, but they are there. Her cheeks are a soft pink. When she wakes, she doesn't want to get up, doesn't want water, doesn't want to watch television, and seems irritated by my efforts to massage her. As I sit next to her, I feel a sense of despair.

It's not easy finding information on when death is imminent – most of the top entries in online searches talk about the last days. *A change in breathing. Lack of interest in food and drink. Feeling very hot or very cold. Mottled skin colour, especially in the extremities. Change in colour of the skin. Rattling, congested-sounding breathing.* Very few talk about the weeks or months leading to death, about gauging how long one might have left to live.

But if truth be told, I don't need the internet to see that Mum hasn't got long to go.

I tell Dennis that I think Mum is reaching the end of her life, watch for his reaction. He is strangely calm.

'At least she won't suffer any more,' he says.

A few days later, when I'm about to head home from another visit to Mum, my friend Fiona rings. She was my hairdresser for many years, before retraining as a nurse. She is Katina's daughter, Mum's compatriot, who'd sung so beautifully at the hospital.

Kindness

Fiona tells me her mum's kidneys and liver are starting to fail, that she is delirious. Fiona knows, as well as I do, that this isn't a good sign.

'Fiona, if it's okay, I'll swing by to see you both.'

'You've got stuff to do. You've just been with your Mum ...'

'Just tell me where she is ...'

When I enter the hospital room, Fiona's Mum raises her head from her delirium to greet me. *Yes, of course she knows who I am.* I give her a kiss, pass on Mum's greetings. She is pleased to see me but is soon distracted. She is agitated, calls out, and Fiona does everything she can to make her comfortable – opens a window, offers her water, tries to get her to eat a spoonful of yoghurt. There is frustration and fear in her movements.

Though Fiona is a nurse, in this room she is a daughter, and there is nothing she can really do to make this better for her mother. The signs of approaching death I've been reading about are clear – the ghostly pallor; feeling extremes of temperature; purple, bloated feet.

I quietly ask Fiona if her mum, who is very religious, has asked for a priest. She says that she is refusing to see one, won't talk about anything to do with dying.

'*Theia*, maybe we can say the *Pater Imon,* the Lord's Prayer, together. I should have concentrated more at Greek school. Let's see if I can remember it,' I joke. She nods.

I start tentatively, '*Pater Imon, oen tis ouranis ...*' Our Father, who art in heaven ...

Theia joins me and then goes off in a clear, confident voice, rising from her delirium, to recite the whole prayer. When she finishes, she looks pleased with herself. *I've still got it,* her expression seems to say. We tell her how impressed we are with her recitation. I tell her I love her, that Mum loves her, that she is a good and kind person. Fiona sits at the end of the bed, weeping quietly.

Fiona's sisters arrive, and a softly spoken doctor comes in, talks about doing more tests on Monday. I leave the room to give them some privacy. In doorways, I see other families milling about their elderly loved ones – a daughter feeding her mother, a grandson holding out a hand to lead his grandfather to bed. Each is a mirror, same but different – all of us trying to do our best for our vulnerable elders. Soon after, Fiona comes out.

'Mum isn't well at all. The doctor won't call it, but I wonder if we should stop the treatment. Just try and make her comfortable …'

'I don't know, Fiona … perhaps listen to your gut. It's not an easy decision to make.' I look Fiona in the eyes. We both know where this is going. 'Maybe talk with your sisters …'

A few days later, Fiona texts to say that her mother died the previous night. That she is sad, but also feels peaceful. Her mum is no longer suffering.

Several days later, I am at Fiona's house, helping with the eulogy. She has pages of notes, feels panicked that she hasn't done enough before the funeral scheduled for later that week.

She reads her notes out as I type them into her laptop. Over a bottle of wine and an oversized packet of potato chips, we craft and add to the eulogy, until we both feel there are enough words to adequately capture who her mother was, to celebrate the life she lived. We manage to hold it together, but when we are finished, we both cry for our mothers – hers who has just gone, and mine who is getting ready to go.

*

It's early October. When I visit Mum, she barely opens her mouth to eat, sleeps for longer each day. She's been moaning more loudly, more regularly, working up to a crescendo on my visits in the afternoons. But her eyes, her eyes are the most upsetting of all. They have become vacant. Pained. Tired. I can't look into them without wanting to wail.

On a recent visit, I'd caught the clinical manager in the reception area. I implored him not to sugar-coat things: if we needed to have a conversation about Mum being in the process of dying sooner than later, then, please, let's do that. I need to get mentally prepared. But he had reassured me they will do what they can to get her weight up, or at least maintain it.

In an email to him, I made suggestions about what Mum seems to enjoy – desserts, juices, water – and how it seems to me that she's in more pain. She can't ask to be moved in her bed, can't ask to be put into her wheelchair or taken off of it.

He promised to get the doctor back, review her analgesia. He noted that if they give her heavier pain medication such as the opioid Endone, it could make her constipated. She has been put on the maximum Panadol, with occasional Endone as backup. Our email exchanges are respectful, forthcoming: I feel we are working together in a bid to make Mum as comfortable as possible. Not for the first time, I'm so grateful this is happening at this aged care home, not the previous one.

Dennis and I keep filling in her food chart dutifully. Her pressure sore has resurfaced and small new ones appear on her feet. Every time I am in, I ask to have her turned. I feel useless and a nuisance. Mum is unfailingly polite to carers, manages a smile sometimes, dutifully allows herself to be changed and turned. I stand in the corner, sometimes outside the door, and hear her moans, try to steel myself. This is not a way to live.

In the day I am competent, focused, but in the night, the dreaded insomnia is rarely far away, and I wake in the small hours of the morning. My thoughts speed ahead, planning for what must be done once Mum has died: photos need to be collated, the priest approached, the cemetery contacted, the funeral director. I can't switch off. My head is on overdrive, constantly.

In my waking moments, I realise that not all of these things need to happen just yet, at least not all at once. Still, over coming days I make sure that all my classes are prepared for the rest of the semester; get up to date with all my marking so that I might pass on my teaching obligations to my colleagues if need be at short notice.

I wake early one morning and write Mum's eulogy, something I've been wanting to do a for a long time. I want to honour Mum with my words, but I feel they are inadequate – how can I possibly summarise Mum's life and her inimitable spirit?

To complicate matters, in the Greek church, the eulogy is only able to be read out by the priest or one of their helpers, not family members. This doesn't always go well – I've been to funerals where the name of the deceased has been read incorrectly, or the priest has fumbled over unfamiliar English words.

I start with the more detailed eulogy I plan to read at the wake. *How does one begin to describe a life? One might start in the sultana fields and olive groves in a small seaside village called Petalidi …*

I write about all the points at which one might start writing about Mum's life: Might it be at her birth, the date of which was not recorded? During her time on the ship to Australia, where the gold coins her father had given her got stolen? Or the time she got run over, potentially ending her life prematurely?

I write that her story might start at any of those points, but for me the story starts and ends with Mum's spirit: *Her body may be gone but her spirit lives on. It lives on in the good deeds that she did for those of us blessed to know her, to call her our mother, our grandmother, our mother-in-law, our sister, our aunty, our friend. It lives on in the memories we have of her and of the way she made us feel. Hers was a beautiful story of how one could be good and kind and generous. For me,* this *is where her story properly begins.*

I don't cry until I write the final words. I feel strangely calm afterwards. I put the draft aside. The next time I look at it, I suspect Mum will no longer be with us.

Though we have been to many Greek funerals, Dennis and I don't really know what religious rituals need to be followed once Mum dies. I remember being in Greece, where the body of an aunt was watched over in an all-night vigil before the funeral, family wailing and lamenting over it. It was primal and comforting. I'd made the same sound in the car on the way to the hospital on learning that my best friend Katerina had died.

Would we need to cleanse Mum's body soon after death like we did for Katerina? What would we need to do to prepare for the funeral?

With the help of a search engine, I'm reminded that there is a service prior to the funeral, called a *trisagion*, which is a hymn evoking God three times. Then there is the funeral service, the burial, and a meal afterwards, known as the *makaria* or mercy meal. I will need to prepare or purchase *koliva*, a memorial dish made of wheat, almonds and dried fruit. There are commemorative services nine days after the funeral, and again after three, six and 12 months. As an observer of other people's mourning, I've often appreciated these markers – it ensures that those who have died are remembered regularly, that the grieving are not forgotten either. But I understand that so much public grieving might be a burden too.

Days later, I text a friend who, coincidently, works at the cemetery where Dad is buried. She looks up the details of Dad's gravesite and reminds me that I am the custodian. I now recall Mum transferring ownership to me just before the lockdowns. She was often worried about Dennis being alone after she died, and that included him being buried on his own. She was not pleased when the cemetery confirmed that Dad's gravesite could only accommodate one more body. On the balance of probabilities, this was likely to be hers. My friend provides the site number, tells me to give it to the funeral director when the time comes.

I bring Mum tetra packs of milk and juices, high calorie desserts. Most of the time she has a spoonful or two. I go from visiting four days a week to five, staying longer to get more meals into her, trying to make sure she is comfortable. Dennis visits on the remaining days, often stays for several hours. We debrief the visits over the phone each time. He seems to be settling down, isn't crying as much. I broach the topic of Mum's funeral, when the time comes, and he is calm, practical. It's clear that he too has done some thinking on it. We make a list of things that will need to be done. We agree about where it will be held, about who to inform and what we need to do. I'm pleased we agree on most things. Mum didn't want us to fight, and though we are very different people, we seem to be capable of honouring her wishes.

When George and Emmanuel visit, they see how emaciated Mum is. Emmanuel places his hands on my shoulders, squeezes. In the car park, he leans over and gives me a hug. I ask him if his black suit pants still fit.

He nods, looks at me evenly. 'It's good you're getting prepared, Mum.'

GIFT #11

Compassion

*I will look into your eyes to see
what is in your heart*

October 2023

Every time I visit Mum, there seems to be less of her. Her once sparkling blue eyes are faded. I can't help but feel her spirit, her very essence, is seeping out of her body.

I speak with the staff in the office and then the clinical manager. I tell them it seems that Mum has given up, that perhaps we need to talk about whether they think she is now actively dying. He seems taken aback by my comments, but if Mum has taught me anything, it's that you should not be shy in talking about death. *It will come for all of us.*

The clinical manager organises another doctor review shortly after. In an email, he confirms that given her wounds aren't healing and her continued weight loss, it is fair to say she was heading towards an 'active palliative pathway', and that they should take measures to keep her as comfortable as possible. The next morning, I go in and speak to him: is he able to give me an indication of how much time Mum might have? He can't say: it could be days, weeks or months. He asks my permission to call the palliative care service attached to the home. When I agree, he says they will be in touch. He asks what we need, and I say

Compassion

I will talk to my brother, to other family members, and will let him know if we need anything. I'm grateful for his kindness and sensitivity – it can't be an easy conversation to have.

Dennis is strangely calm when I tell him. We sit together all day beside Mum, who dips in and out of sleep. Later that evening, he goes home. That night, as I am ready to go home, an older carer comes by, takes a shrewd look at Mum.

She says gently, 'I think it will happen quickly.'

I'm surprised, pleased at her honesty. I lay down on the mat beside Mum's bed. I'm not letting her do this alone.

*

The next day, nothing has changed. I text and call several people who have been close to Mum and our family. It's not long before family and friends congregate in Mum's room, in the corridors, outside in the courtyard. Emmanuel sits beside her all day, holding her hand. Her nieces and their children sit on the floor beside her bed. Dolores calls to speak to her over the phone from overseas, frustrated and sad that she can't be here. She's organised the next flight home, won't hear of staying any longer. Dennis seems calm, buoyed by the support of family. Mum looks a little bewildered by all the activity, but seems calm. She dips in and out of sleep.

Later that afternoon, I tell Mum that the priest is visiting the care home, that he will come by her room. It's hard to tell if she understands me but she doesn't appear distressed.

The priest, whose number I had put into my phone for just such an occasion, picks up on the first ring. I explain in halting Greek that Mum is dying, and could he please come and read a prayer?

He answers in English, sympathetic. 'Is she still conscious?'

'Yes,' I say.

He tells me he is unwell, but he will ask his assistant priest to call me. The young priest calls, and shortly afterwards, a very tall, solidly built young man clad in his black vestments meets me in the foyer. We dispense with the fiddly check in-process – there is a sense of urgency. As we enter the lounge, one of the Greek residents raises her hand to call him over. When she eyes the black bag, her hand falls, her face clouded with concern. She knows why the priest is here.

The priest carefully unpacks his little black suitcase as if he is about to perform surgery – a stole carefully laid over Mum's bed, a prayer read over her, and a small vial of wine poured into a container given to her on a petite gold spoon. Mum looks up at his immense height, her concentration lapsing only to look around the room at the people around her bed. She looks back at him. Takes it all in. *What does this mean? Am I dying?* She knows. The worry about the process. The wormhole. It's happening.

After a short prayer, the priest downs the rest of the wine, carefully wipes the spoon and packs up. I follow him out, try to press some money into his hand. He waves it aside.

'I don't want to be paid. Give it to someone who needs a meal.'

Compassion

*

'Cous, I think it's happening. I don't want to alarm you. But I know you want to be here ...'

I'd called my cousin Kathy in the small hours of Saturday morning, and she'd come in soon after. She's made it clear to me that she wanted to be there when Mum died. She'd often chided Mum for sending her away from Dad's deathbed to buy rusks and coffee to feed the many mourners who would visit. There was no way she was going to miss being there for Mum when she died.

Mum's breathing is laboured, and we are like little girls once again – nervous, morbidly excited at being left alone with big responsibility. Where once it was being left alone to cook and look after her younger siblings, now it is about being with Mum as she's dying. We ring Dim, describe Mum's breathing to her. Might we be hearing the death rattle? She doesn't think so.

We sit beside Mum, fear that if we head out for even just a few minutes to go to the toilet, or grab a coffee, we might miss her last minutes. I can't help but think of the circularity of things. Once Kathy and I walked arm in arm at dinner dances, dressed in matching dresses that Mum had sewn for us. As a young woman, I attended the births of her daughters – encouraging her to *push, push*. Seeing her girls being born felt miraculous on a spiritual level beyond compare. Now we sit with Mum, whisper in her ear that it's okay to leave, play her Greek liturgy, massage her hands and feet.

Mum gets through the night. More people come to visit the next day – cousins Dim and Georgia, and their girls, my cousin Jorge, Mum's sister Voula and my cousin Christine. The room feels like a cocoon, and we dip in and out of stories all day.

That night, Kathy and I sit either side of Mum. We are unable to sleep and tell more stories. Kathy vividly remembers saying goodbye to Mum at the bus stop when our family were leaving Narrandera, says it broke her heart. Years later, their family would join us in Melbourne, and it felt as if we just took up where we had left off. I know that Mum has been a big influence on the woman Kathy has become. It's obvious in the way she shares her home, her generous table, her arms always open, working hard for the ones she loves.

I share the stories that I have written about Mum, about finding the jewellery box amongst her things. Kathy says her Mum had the same one, that she would have liked to keep it, but it was thrown away. I vow to gift her Mum's, perhaps with a piece of her jewellery as a memento. We reflect on the many conversations we have had about what life might be like without Mum in it. *And now it's happening.*

The next day, Kathy looks exhausted and finally goes home. It could be a while yet before Mum leaves us.

*

Compassion

The sky is dark, and the stars feel surprisingly near. I walk the dark suburban path, holding Mum's bunched up blanket close to my chest. It's been on her bed these past few months, close to her body, and I cling to it as if I'm clinging to her. *I don't want you to leave. I don't want to let you go.*

A wail bursts from my gut and chest and out of my mouth, a primal, wrenching sound. It cuts through the darkness, forming bursts of white mist. Even though the sound is terrible, I know it needs to come out, and I let it. I'm grateful that the care home abuts quiet paths and old orchards, that there is no one to see a grief-crazed, sleep-deprived woman wailing into the night.

Five days after it was declared that Mum was dying, she is still clinging on. I've been with her constantly, showering in her bathroom, sleeping for a few hours each night on the chair beside her bed. One of the personal carers tells me that not many people stay by the bedside as I have done. That perhaps I need to get some rest at home. Her words are firm but kind.

I've resisted leaving Mum's side up until now, but I'm starting to feel unhinged with fatigue and grief. And part of me wonders whether she might not go while I'm there. George comes in. I blabber indecisively. He sends me to the car so I might get some rest. He sits with Mum; says he will ring me if anything changes. In the car, I'm hyped, can't nap. Instead, I walk around the block, clinging to Mum's blanket, trying to avoid the cracks on the footpath, and keep wailing into the night. I realise I need to say goodbye. I need to go home and prepare for the fact that next time I see her, Mum might have already wriggled through the wormhole.

I need to let you go. I need to let you go.

*

The next day, I come in at 6 am, and Mum is still breathing. The personal carer who delivered sandwiches on the first day, quietly delivers more, along with a cup of tea. His eyes are sympathetic – he understands how difficult this is. I ask if I can give him a hug to thank him for his kindness. I give him a thank you card, a small gift. Another worker comes in, and she turns her head away from me, swats at tears. She apologises for getting upset, asks when Mum became palliative. I tell her there is no need to apologise. I'm moved by her tears. I've connected with her, and she with Mum. I give her a hug too and pass her a card and gift to say thanks. I'm so glad these workers, who are both older and have been in this line of work for a long time, haven't lost their humanity.

George joins me later that morning, and Mum surprises us with a few hours of her lucid attention: she smiles wryly at George when he brings in more supplies; we look together at photos. Later, she mumbles something about sewing, that I should keep sewing. I promise her I will.

The following day, Mum is still battling. She is not drinking, and I wet her lips with a cotton stick to keep her comfortable.

Compassion

Family friends come by, read a prayer over Mum. George goes home after sitting with us all day, but around 9 pm, the sounds that Mum is making have changed, and I call him back in. He brings more food: moussaka, rice pudding, potato chips, a thermos of tea and a water bottle. Mum dips in and out of sleep, but her breathing is laboured, gurgling. She is on four-hourly morphine, has been given medication to allay agitation. We are told we can call the care staff at any time during the night, but they largely leave us in the quiet twilight of the room. The palliative care service had called earlier today: *could they do anything to help?* I'd said we were doing as well as could be expected, that we didn't need anything at this stage.

Mum settles into a fitful sleep, and I send George home. I should sleep but am restless. I crack open the chips, send messages back and forth to Dolores, who has just said a teary goodbye to her travel companion, is waiting at the airport for her flight. In the small hours of the night, I tell her I have just eaten a family-size packet of chips. She says I deserve to eat a million packets of chips. Her words are like an anchor in the murky darkness of the room.

At around 4 that morning, Mum's breathing becomes even more laboured. She is trying to cough but hasn't the strength. She sounds like she is drowning in her own fluids. I press the button beside Mum's bed, and the nurse and a carer come in to discuss what should be done. I step outside into the foyer. I've tried to be strong for Mum, to stand by her through everything, but this feels like too much. A resident is sitting quietly in the foyer. There are dim lights at the nurse's station, the hum of air conditioning. I pace it out, try to take deep, slow breaths so that I might get through this.

When I return to the room, the nurse says they will ask the doctor, who will be coming in at 6 am, to organise two-hourly morphine. The nurse touches Mum on the way out, says, 'It's okay to let go, Chrisoula. Why are you holding on so hard?'

Once more drugs have been organised for Mum, and I know George will be awake, I call him to come in. Mum is dying, and I don't want to do this alone.

*

Early that morning, Kathy comes in with coffee and toast. George arrives soon after with more food, and Dim shortly after that. I ring Dennis – I tell him that it seems like Mum might be passing away today. Does he want to be here? He says he doesn't want to – *can't* – be there. I say that this is okay, that he must do what feels right.

Dim sits at Mum's feet. Kathy takes one of Mum's hands, George the other, and I sit beside Mum's head, whisper gentle words into her ear: *You are safe. Join your father. It's his naming day today. Dimitri. A beautiful name for a beautiful man. Kind and generous, just like you,* Mamma mou. *It's okay to go to him. You can go.*

Compassion

It feels like a meditation of sorts, words and Greek liturgy and touch working together. There are no stories today. Everything we do is about helping Mum along.

Dim watches Mum's pulse, reports when it stops. Kathy notes the time: a little after 11. There are no more words, no sounds, no breath. Mum's body is still here, her hands in our hands, but she is gone.

GIFT #12

Spirit

I will try to look up when I am down

October 2023

I'm still reeling from Mum's death yesterday. I have flashbacks of waiting for the doctor to confirm she had died, sitting with her still body; the undertakers coming and placing her on a trolley, covering her body with a silken, embroidered cloth; the quiet walk through the communal area of the home; and all the staff standing, sombre, hands crossed in front of their bodies; my cousins, George and me behind them. It was strangely soothing, peaceful. It felt like a respectful way to say our goodbyes.

Afterwards, I had asked staff to keep Mum's custom wheelchair. I'd been packing her things through the night, not knowing what else to do. These we took to the car. Mum has spent five months in this home. Though it was so hard watching Mum's decline, I'm grateful to the home for providing us with such a dignified environment, for their sensitive care of her. For *seeing* her.

Dennis had been waiting at home to hear news. I'd not wanted to tell him over the phone, had driven over to his house to tell him in person. He'd looked stricken but kept repeating,

'At least she's at peace now.' We'd sat together, talking and preparing for what would come next: planning for her funeral.

*

This evening, one day after Mum died, we are meeting with the funeral director at Mum's home. When he comes to the door, I see he is a dapper-looking man, suited up with a black bag, a little like the priest. He says his condolences, and we make small talk – he's had two funerals today. His demeanour is sympathetic, but professional. We tell him we have decided on our preferred church. That Mum has an existing plot. That we want to have a wake afterwards at the church. And that we would like to have the funeral by next Thursday if possible – so that both our children can be there. Dolores is coming home from overseas tomorrow, and Emmanuel is leaving for a trip to Vietnam the following week.

The funeral director looks unsure.

'If you want a notice to go in the Greek paper, it will have to be Monday for a Thursday funeral. I would need to confirm with the priest, and the cemetery, to see if they can book it in. Given the cemetery office is closed for the weekend, that's not going to be possible …'

I tell him I can call on a friend at the cemetery. He waits while I ring her.

'Um, Robyn, I wonder if I can ask a favour …'

She says she will call me back once she has made some calls – someone will need to check the roster, see if there is availability.

In the meantime, the funeral director walks us through various choices – a casket versus coffin. He explains that coffins are tapered at the ends, are generally smaller. He shows us some photos from a folder.

'Is Mum a larger lady?' he asks delicately.

'No, not in recent years.'

'It might feel like she's swimming in the casket.'

A coffin it is.

Next, we look at photos of coffins, ranging from those priced in the many thousands of dollars, to a simple wooden box. Dennis and I quickly narrow it down to a mid-range coffin that is elegant but not too ostentatious.

We need to decide if we want a keepsake card. Dennis is keen, but I'm not sure it's necessary, wonder if we can just do our own. I think of the photos that still need to be chosen, the eulogy bedded down, the visitors that will be dropping in, booking the hall and deciding on catering … We should let the funeral company deal with the card.

While we are waiting for Robyn to ring back, we talk about the life of a funeral director. How long he's been in the business, how he started.

'Do you enjoy the job?'

'It's interesting. You meet all sorts of people. But the hours are long ... you don't have a life. I always seem to be late for dinner.' He smiles wryly. *What can you do?*

I'm not surprised at how busy he is – the Greek paper is filled each week with more and more people dying from my parents' generation. And disturbingly, people in their fifties and sixties.

When Robyn hasn't called back, we let the funeral director get home to his dinner. He tells us to ring him at any time once availability at the cemetery has been confirmed.

*

The next morning, George and I pick Dolores up from the airport. It's been nearly three months since we've seen her. The reunion is bittersweet – what should be a time of sharing and excitement after her first independent trip overseas is underpinned by sadness – she missed her yiayia's death and has flown back to find us in mourning. At home, we enjoy a quiet meal, a bit of respite before the chaos of the next week begins.

In the afternoon there are phone calls back and forth – our preferred date for the funeral is set. Family friends drop in to pay their respects. We generate a task list: informing people about the *trisagion* the day before the funeral, and the funeral; deciding on words and photos for the funeral notice and memorial card; collating photos for the wake and organising who will speak;

dropping off Mum's clothes to the funeral parlour; finalising the eulogy.

I dig out the draft I wrote some weeks ago, the version I will read at the wake. I read it over, add to it. I ask George and Dolores to review it, check some small details with my cousins. Though mere words will never do Mum's spirit justice, I'm happy with it. Now, what words to write for the priest to read out? These will have to wait, as there are texts and phone calls to respond to: people wanting to visit as per Greek tradition – sitting with the bereaved, telling stories, remembering the deceased over black coffee and unsweetened rusks. I tell them we will be at Mum's house tomorrow afternoon, sorting through photos – they can come and help us take a trip down memory lane together – otherwise they will find us at home.

I realise that, while Mum's clothes are ready to be taken to the funeral parlour, I can't find the shoes and the silken underclothes she had made me pack all that time ago. I know her feet will be covered, but hear her voice echoing in my ears: *Don't forget the shoes!* I ring my niece Sophia, who is at the shops. She says she will buy shoes, along with arranging and dropping off some thank you cakes to the aged care home. I make a trip to the shops to buy Mum undergarments. I drop all these things off to the funeral home.

The next morning, I attend church to see if I can catch the priest to confirm the details of the funeral service, and the wake in the church hall afterwards.

Spirit

At church, I'm not prepared for the emotional tsunami of seeing so many women – white-haired, dark-clad, stooped – that remind me of Mum. *How is it that these women are here and my mother is not?* As soon as I light my candle, I make my way to a corner of the packed church to sob, hoping no one notices.

At the end of the service, an older woman who had formed a connection with Mum when they were each picking up their grandkids at school many years ago, asks how Mum is. I tell her she died only days ago, and the tears start again. She and those around her look at me sympathetically, offer their condolences. The familiarity of the words repeated when someone dies – *Theos sihoresti*, May God forgive her; *Zoi se esas*, Life to you – is comforting.

I make my way up to the nave, where the priest warmly greets me, offers his condolences. He has a longstanding relationship with our family: he was Mum's boss when she was sewing nighties many years ago. When it became clear that the manufacturing industry was dying, he'd retrained as a priest, following in his own father's footsteps. Mum had always encouraged him to follow the vocation, but he was resistant at that time.

During services, he is at time brusque with his elderly parishioners, has a decidedly dark sense of humour. He would often good-naturedly tell Mum off for being impatient when he was running late to bless Dad's grave. And she would tease him about not paying her enough when she sewed for him.

He confirms that the funeral director has been in touch, that the service is locked in.

'Have you booked the church hall for the wake?' he says.

'I didn't know I had to. I thought the funeral director took care of it.'

He says that it's up to us and calls over to a grey-haired man.

'Dimitri, Spiridoula here needs help with the hall for next Thursday. Look after her, she's from our parts of Greece!'

I smile – even after more than half a century of Greeks being in Australia, some things never change – and follow Dimitri out to the area behind the church. He walks me through the two church halls, talks about the number of tables and chairs needed, about costs and logistics.

'Have you booked catering?' he says.

'Isn't that part of the hall booking?'

'No, we don't organise that. The guy you need to speak to about it is in Greece … I'll try and dig up some numbers for you.'

How to find a caterer for more than 100 people with fewer than four days to go before the funeral? It's yet another thing to do.

On the way out, I bump into the priest.

'All okay, Spiridoula?'

'Yes, thank you.' I look him in the eyes. 'You'll look after Mum, make sure she goes straight up?!'

I'm not sure how he's going to take it, whether he will berate me for blasphemy, but he meets my gaze, laughs.

'Don't worry. I'll use extra holy water!'

I smile at his retreating back, black robes flapping. *We're going to get through this.*

*

A few days before the funeral, I still have to write the words the priest will read out about Mum in church. I recall doing the same for Dad. For his eulogy, I used Cavafy's beautiful poem 'Ithaka' to frame the words. The choice was perfect for Dad. Once I'd decided on it, the words had flown out onto the page almost fully formed.

Now, I need to sit down, concentrate my energies at this terribly sad time, to write words that will do Mum justice. But my hands lie still, paralysed by the enormity of the task. I try to think about her before she lay prone in her bed, before her diagnosis, before she lost her words …

I think of your name, *Mamma mou.* Chrisoula. *The golden one.*

I see your face light up when you open the door to your home, welcoming us in.

I imagine your hands, filling our plates with home-made chips. '*Faye, faye!* Eat, eat!'

I hear your laughter, tinkling, even in your darkest moments.

And your eyes. Your eyes. Kind, cheeky and wise. I look inside their blue depths, and they fill me with energy and love.

All I have to do is think of your voice, your touch, your gaze – through these you gave us so many golden gifts, *Mamma mou*. You showed us what it was like to feel welcome around a table. How to throw open one's doors, arms and heart to let people in. How to work hard for those you love. How to make things happen, gently but persistently, by being kind.

You have been giving me these gifts my whole life, even when I didn't realise it. Perhaps I didn't appreciate them enough in the past, but I know now how precious they are, how lucky I am to have them. I've tried to use them as best I could to look after you in your time of greatest need.

I imagine you passing these gifts on to me. They are still warm with your touch. They sparkle with your intention, shine with your love and your golden spirit. I think of how I might put them to good use, as you have done so often in the past.

Once the gifts are in my hands, their golden energy flows through me, and words pour out and onto the page …

*

Dolores wants to speak at her yiayia's wake. I remind her several times that she needs to get some words down, and she tells me she hasn't forgotten – she will do it when she is ready.

The day before the funeral, she passes her laptop across to me, asks me to read over what she has written. When I finish,

Spirit

I tell her through tears that her words are perfect. I wouldn't change a single thing.

> My yiayia is unlike anyone I've ever known.
>
> She never had a bad word to say about anyone, and no one had a bad word to say about her.
>
> She welcomes us (and anyone else we happen to drag along) into her house with open arms, cheeky words, and a table brimming with food.
>
> She has raised a good proportion of the people in this room, whether they are her own children or not, and has done so with unbelievable levels of kindness, responsibility and selflessness.
>
> She always puts others before herself, making sure that everyone else is fed and comfortable before she even sits down.
>
> Even in her last months and weeks and days and moments, she was polite to a fault and expressed nothing but positivity and quiet acceptance. But, as strong as she was during this time, this is not how I will remember her.
>
> Instead, I will remember her famous *tyganites patates*, or fried potatoes. Every time we come over for dinner, she makes them for our family because she knows how much Emmanuel and I love them. We step through her front door and make a beeline to the stove, where a heap of warm *tyganites patates* is always sitting in a '70s-style tan and

cream Tupperware container. We eat them one after the other, and Mum tuts that we won't have any room left over for dinner, but Yiayia just smiles and says, not to worry, there are more coming.

I will remember her post-dinner money-giving ritual. At the end of the night, as we are rounding up the bottles of milk and packets of toilet paper that Yiayia is sending home with us, she slips quietly away to the cupboard in the hallway and retrieves her peeling leather wallet. She pulls out a 20-dollar note, crushes it into my hand, and says: "Don't tell your mother." She has been doing this for as long as I can remember. I tell her, "Yiayia, I don't need it. I'm an adult now. I'm making my own money." She frowns and fusses and tells me this is different because it's from her and that it makes her happy because she's helping her grandchildren. I've discovered over the years that fighting her is futile, so I give her a kiss on the cheek and say, "Okay, Yiayia. Thank you."

I will remember her garden. It's a warm spring day and she calls Dad out from the house to come look at her tomatoes. He speaks in broken Greek to her, expressing his awe at her thriving plants and asking her for tips. You can tell she is chuffed. Then she goes into the bungalow and fetches an old doona. We roll it out onto the grass and lie under her orange trees, watching the sun filter through leaves and slapping the ants that crawl onto our arms.

Yiayia keeps trying to get up, to chop us fruit or make us coffee, and Mum keeps pulling her back down, telling her to relax for once. But the truth is that Yiayia is happiest when she is doing things for the people she loves, because that's just the kind of person she is.

The words I've spoken today are in the present tense. They were in the present tense when they were in my head, and I decided to write them down this way too. They're in the present tense because, though Yiayia is gone, the person she was is still very much alive. Her life and legacy have touched so many people both inside and outside her family, and she will live on through memories and stories and bloodlines.

Yiayia, I love you, and miss you already, but I know you're in a better place now, probably having a beer with Pappou up there somewhere. Thank you for everything you have done for me and our family. We will never forget you.

The morning of the funeral arrives. I lay the same black dress I have worn to so many funerals onto the bed, dark stockings, heels I bought in Greece many years ago. The ironing board is out for the last-minute shirt pressings. As mandated by tradition, oil and wine and homemade bread, *prosforo,* have been set aside for the church service. There is nothing more to be done.

At church, we file into the front pews. The coffin is brought in and the lid opened as per tradition. The chanting, the incense is comforting in its familiarity. *Aionia I mnimi, Aionia I mnimi* is chanted over and over. Eternal be her memory, eternal be her memory. The priest reads the words I have prepared in Greek, and a younger one reads them in English.

>Chrisoula was her name, from the Greek word χρυσο, meaning 'gold'.
>
>Chrisoula welcomed you to her door with an open heart and open arms, no matter the time of day or night.
>
>She always asked you to sit at her table and shared whatever she had, even when she didn't have much.
>
>She always had a warm hug ready when you needed it.
>
>She listened to your problems, even when she had many of her own.
>
>She made you feel that even if your heart was heavy, there was always something to laugh about.
>
>She believed that if you had a good word to say to someone, one that would make them walk a little straighter, you should say it.
>
>She taught you that if someone was down, and if you could help them, you should.
>
>She showed you that actions were just as important as words.
>
>She showed you that with hard work, and focusing on the ones you love, you could achieve a lot of things.
>
>She looked straight into your eyes, and often knew what was in your heart.

Spirit

She believed that if you could take joy from small pleasures, you should embrace that joy wholeheartedly.

She believed that if you were down, there was only one way to go – and that was up.

She gave us many golden gifts. Our hope is that these will live on in whomever was lucky enough to receive them.

It is with great sorrow that we farewell our beloved Chrisoula, but we take heart that her wonderful spirit lives on inside us.

Only at the end of the service do I see how many people have come to commemorate Mum and to support us. As they file past our family, offering their condolences, I am overwhelmed by the sheer number of people: old family friends, neighbours, colleagues and friends of ours, and several people I don't recognise. I worry that we haven't catered for enough people, make a mental note to ring the caterer on the way to the cemetery, warn her there may be more than anticipated.

At the cemetery, the priest reads a prayer over the grave, and the coffin is slowly lowered into the ground. I wail. *I'm not ready to let you go, I'm not ready to let you go.* Hands surround me, hold me, lead me away. Later, when most mourners have left for the church hall, I go back, look down into the hole where Mum's coffin rests on top of the concrete slab that holds Dad's remains below it. A family friend looks at me with concern – *will there be more hysterics?* – but I'm now calm. Dennis and I and a few family friends stand around, gently joking about Mum and Dad's reunion. Will it be amicable? They've been nearly 20 years apart – they will have to get used to each other again.

The wake passes in a flurry of activity – there is a meal, a slideshow of photos, silent and powerful, and then I, and Dolores speak. Dolores gets through her speech – pausing in the middle to compose herself.

'Be strong, Dolores!' my frail father-in-law calls out. The room breaks out in laughter, and Dolores continues.

Finally, my niece Sophia speaks. She remembers her yiayia looking after her while her parents were working. Her yiayia and pappou taught her so many things, from learning to plant tomatoes, to how to cross herself in church, to how to buy a ticket on the bus, to how to barter with shop owners: 'Cash, dahling!' They taught her how to have a home where people feel welcome. And how to have a listening ear, but a 'mouth that bites back when need be'. She is going to miss many things about her yiayia, but most of all, her response when she would say the words, 'Yiayia, I love you.' And Mum would always respond: *'Ego na theis.'* You should see how much *I* love you.

Sophia shares a video reel and photos: of her dancing with Mum at her wedding, Mum opening the door and being surprised and overjoyed to see her, Mum cuddling Sophia's new baby, Mum and Dad giving each other a kiss. It feels so strange to see Mum up on the screen so alive and well.

Spirit

As soon as the reel is over, mourners start saying goodbye: some have to pick up grandkids from school, others need to get back to elderly partners.

It's over. It feels final, but also surreal. *Is Mum* really *gone? And what now?*

*

My best friend Katerina died over a decade ago after battling with cancer for several years, my father died nearly 20 years ago – I'm no stranger to people close to me dying. I know that grief can creep up on you from behind, wash right over you like a tsunami when you least expect it. I tell myself that over the past few years we've been grieving many incremental losses. *Missing the daily phone call with Mum. Missing her opening her door to her house. Missing being able to have a conversation that made sense.* We have had time to get used to her demise. Hopefully this time it won't hit so hard. I know what to expect.

Mum's picture, the one we put in the paper, keeps us company at the dinner table when we eat, or do the morning crossword. It's surrounded by several vases of flowers, bunches of which kept arriving for many days after Mum died. They take up half the table, so that we have to squish up around them when we have meals. I speak to her, say good morning when I come into the room, make sure to include her in our 'cheers' at the start of a meal. The flowers that arrived soon after she died wilt and brown, shedding pollen all over the table, and must be thrown out. I save just a few stems to put in a single vase. I'm thinking about transience as I wash the vases. *The flowers were beautiful. They will die. We will replace them with new flowers from the garden. And so it goes.*

The cemetery where she is buried is only a 15-minute walk from our house. It's reassuring knowing she is so close.

The next morning, George and I walk there. A sheet of particle board and a heavy grate cover the grave, with several bunches of flowers atop it. The stone hasn't yet been replaced over the tomb.

'You're with Dad. I know he'll be happy to see you,' I tell her. As if he can 'see' now. Still, it's reassuring.

George agrees. 'They've been apart a long time.'

We light the candle and incense. The pungent smell of smoke, its sweet undertone of rose, wafts across the other graves. I splash some water on the wreaths sent by my cousins' families, take one last look at the grave, admire the flowers that fill the bucket, say goodbye for now.

The following day, I come with my brother. The stone has been set back on the tomb, stuck on with a thick clear sealant that reminds me of shower recesses. I watch Dennis for signs of distress, but his face is in repose, his eyes dry. There's been a certain shift in his demeanour since Mum died. Relief. *She is no longer in pain. He can finally start getting on with his life.*

Spirit

We both agree that nothing feels quite real about this. *Light the candle and incense. Wash the grave down. Throw out dying flowers. Wash our hands.* The physicality of the tasks is reassuring – at least we can still *do* something for her and Dad. All the while, we talk about the other people buried here. Dennis and I reflect that many in Mum's neighbourhood have died, that there are more dead than living.

Back home, I know that I will need to put the sympathy cards away, work out what to do with the last of her clothes, the miscellany in her handbag. I've shifted these things from the car to the laundry, to the bed, and now back again. I'll deal with them when I've finished marking assignments, helped Dennis with some paperwork, finally submitted my tax return …

*

I wake early, at long last having a free day ahead of me. The past few weeks have passed in a blur. I've returned to teaching. The assignments that piled up during my absence have been marked. The nine-day commemorative service at the church attended. The dust has finally settled. This is as good a time as any to make some decisions about a few of Mum's things. I find a large gift box at the top of a cupboard. I can put the small stuff in there so that it's safe.

First go the sympathy cards. I'm not sure if I should respond to each individually, send a thank you note, but the task seems overwhelming, and I don't have most people's addresses. After posting about Mum's death on Facebook, dozens upon dozens of sympathy messages had poured in. There were so many text messages and phone calls in the days and weeks after. I've done my best to respond to each soon after it came in, but there's a prick of anxiety. Have I missed anyone? I consider reading the cards again, but that will get me teared up even before I've started. *Not yet.* In the box they go.

I'd taken most of the clothes she wore in the care home to the op shop – functional tracksuits and tops that were easy to slide on, things that had been purchased or received as gifts in the past year. I've kept three summer frocks that Mum wore when she first went into care. All are black but with different patterns: little white flowers, repeated circles and geometric designs. For many years they've been Mum's summer staple – easy to throw on, taking no time at all to hand wash in the laundry trough each night, quick to dry overnight, and they didn't need ironing – they were practical like Mum herself. I pick them up slowly, hoping they smell of her. There's a whiff of laundry powder, a metallic undertone. They've been through the industrial wash at the care home, her familiar smell stripped out of them.

I press the fabric against my nose. I'm overwhelmed by the desire to hold her after she's been in the garden, envelop her in my arms and take in her earthy smell. Take *her* in. I'll never be able to do this again. Tears prick, and I will them not to start.

I place the frocks in the box. It would be sensible to cull them down to one, but I can't bring myself to do it.

There are several combs and brushes. One still has her grey hairs on it. I thought I'd done everything I needed to do to avoid regret down the track, but why didn't I cut some of her hair, perhaps to make little lockets for family as they did in Victorian times? It might seem morbid, but now I get the sentiment. I put the brush with the hair, without cleaning it, on top of the frocks.

Next, I pick up her bag. In it is a prayer book, her wallet, a tissue, two copies of the photo we chose for her grave, and the funeral notice, which Dennis has laminated for me.

I pull out the wallet, look inside. There are some notes. *Always have cash on you.* Her Centrelink and Medicare card. *Do I need to let government departments know she's passed away?* And a fist full of coins. *The coins she always banked up for church.* She won't be using these anymore. The tears I've been holding back start in earnest.

I put the wallet and tissue back, am about to place the whole bag into the box when I see something glinting at the bottom. It's a filigreed brooch, one I thought looked gauche when I was younger. It's made up of curlicued gold leaves, delicately and intricately engraved. I pin it to my chest.

The box is overfull now. Not much has been culled. The lid doesn't close. I put it aside in our bedroom. Place her blanket on top, the book that people signed at her funeral. This too I can't yet bear to open. My big pile spread across the laundry bench has turned into a smaller, more contained one. Still, it's yet another step. *Ride the waves. Take your time. There's no rush.*

The rest of the day is spent cleaning the shower, dusting cobwebs off the windows and eaves, wiping the kitchen floor on hands and knees. This is a long-overdue clean. In a few weeks' time, guests will arrive to commemorate the passing of 40 days after Mum's death. But if I'm honest, I'm trying to scrub my sadness away, pour it out with the dirty mop water, swipe at it with each cobweb that disappears. I can't bring myself to take the filigreed brooch off, though I fear it may get damaged.

At the end of the night, when the house is gleaming like it hasn't done for several months, I place the brooch in a small bowl beside my bed that holds Mum's earrings and her crucifix. More things to decide what to do with. But for now, they are close to me while I sleep.

*

My chest hurts. It feels like a tight pulling pain. It comes when I walk. When I do an exercise class. Sometimes when I'm sitting still.

My doctor listens to my symptoms, looks concerned. He talks about the need to rule out the possibility of angina. Sends me for a stress echocardiogram, an ultrasound that tests heart function before and after walking fast on a treadmill. He tells me it doesn't hurt. He asks me to find out when the results will be sent to him, to make a phone appointment to discuss them with him soon after.

At the consultation I'm asked to strip down from the waist up, and the attendant uses a little abrasive pad that feels like sandpaper, and gel afterwards, to attach ECG electrodes over my chest. She talks me through, and I make awkward jokes to distract myself from the fact she has to shift my breasts to get the electrodes on. But she's a pro, and before I know it, I'm on the table and she's taking images of my heart as she rolls the ultrasound probe over my sternum, to the side of my chest. I angle my head to watch what comes up on the screen.

There's a little flap dangling back and forth – likely a valve between each of the heart chambers. It looks like a little penis. I stifle the urge to laugh, think of how Mum could find humour in almost every situation. But I'm sobered by the thought that this tiny piece of flesh might be working ineffectively, perhaps not closing over properly. I think wryly that it would be terribly unfair, now that I am no longer caring for Mum, that my own health should take a downward turn.

After running on the treadmill and hopping back on the table as quickly as I can to measure my heart function after exercise, the radiographer tells me that the results are normal. The flaccid-looking thing is clearly doing exactly what it's supposed to do.

When I meet with my GP a few days later, he tells me I tolerated exercise quite well. That my blood pressure and heart rate were normal both before and after exercise for someone of my age.

'I'm wondering then if it's not physical. Maybe this is a bit about anxiety,' I say. I've been talking with George, who had similar symptoms a few years back during the height of the lockdowns when he was going through the worst of his experiences with his parents.

'Well, I've just finished having this very same talk with another of my patients. What's been going on that might make you say that?'

'Well, I've just come out of this intense period of caring for, and then losing, Mum. Things are finally settling down ...'

He talks me through the fact that it may be time to start looking after myself, and of the need to look forward. I tell him I will do my best.

The heart pain has scared me. It's a reminder that time is precious, and that I need to appreciate the small daily joys – eating a meal around the table, playing a silly game after dinner, going for a walk with dear friends, bantering with my daughter as we fold the clothes, laughing at George's 'dad' jokes. I need to reconnect with the beautiful things, and people, in my life. I'm trying, but my heart feels heavy.

It's been just on five months since Mum died. Though sadness still clings to me like a second skin, I've found rituals are helping me deal with my grief. *Lighting a candle in front of Mum's photo, saying good morning and goodnight to her. Visiting her grave whenever I feel the need. Spending time with extended family and friends who loved her. Attending church at key milestone dates, having the priest bless her grave. Writing about her, keeping her alive on the page.* It's been helpful to talk and laugh and cry and reminisce.

Dennis and I have been spending a lot of time together. We have lunch each week on the porch at Dennis's house, or at a Vietnamese restaurant I used to frequent with Mum. He regularly comes to our house for dinner. I quietly admire my quirky brother: looking after Mum, and dealing with Mum's death, has brought us closer together. He often comes up with wise words out of the blue. The other day, he'd said, 'Even the most horrible person has something good in them. You just have to listen to their story.'

We've met with the lawyer to start the ball rolling to transfer the ownership of Mum's home and to close off her bank account. We start the process to upgrade the gravesite with new lettering adding Mum's name and making some other changes that she would have liked to make herself after Dad died. We've talked about what we want to do with Mum's home, what is possible. We decide that we can't afford to keep it, that Dennis might move to somewhere smaller, more manageable. This also suits our family, as we are not planning to move from our home in the near future, would like to help our own children with a home purchase down the track. Though I desperately want to honour Mum's wishes, building something on her property is too hard, too expensive. These plans are not just about what we want to do now, but about where we see ourselves living in the future. There is some comfort in looking forward. Still, Dennis and I agree that the saddest moment will be when we turn the key to Mum's home for the last time.

While it feels wrong to talk about Mum's home in legal and financial ways, I'm grateful that Dennis and I are having sensible conversations. That we are not fighting. I know this is not always the case with siblings, that death has a way of bringing up old hurts. I am grateful that Mum and Dad showed us how to care and how to love. Mum worked hard for us, was keen for us to be provided for. I am grateful that settling Mum's estate is relatively straightforward. I can't help but think that even in death, she made it easy for us.

Though things have slowed right down, and I am no longer rushing from care home to Mum's home, to ours and to work, sleep still eludes me. I obsess in the night about what I might have done differently. *Could I have spent more time with Mum before she got really unwell? Should I have acted earlier to get her into care so that we could have avoided her breaking her hip? How might we have prevented her from being in so much pain in the last months of her life?*

I tell myself I tried my best. I did what I could, what felt right at the time. I've worked hard to look after Mum, after Dennis, after my own family and myself so that I could keep going. During the day, I talk myself down, but in the night, I torture myself with the what-ifs. *If I'd acted earlier, would she still be alive now?*

I try to process things, write out the angst, untangle the pain as if unravelling the messy threads in the drawer of Mum's sewing machine. Words fly onto the page in a fat, guilty mess. In the end, I get to the bottom of my heart pain.

I just wanted more of you, Mamma mou.

Epilogue

July 2024

Mamma mou,

We are in the thick of Melbourne winter. You have been gone now for nine months. In the backyard of your home, your garden beds are covered in weeds, but your mandarin tree is heavy with fruit. I pick some every time I come here, give them to family and friends – even to the people that came to collect some of your things from the nature strip.

Dennis is now settled in a brand-new home that's far too big for one man and too far away from our own home. While I worry for him, just as you did, he loves it, looks forward to returning to it when we have spent time together. Though you would have been disappointed that we aren't living next door to each other, you always did like new homes. You would be proud of how Dennis is managing to run a household on his own. I ring him every day; see him regularly. We talk often of the gifts you gave us that made us who we are, that have made our lives more comfortable.

Packing up your home has been heartbreaking, *Mamma mou*. What to do with all those embroidered tablecloths you collected over the years? All those crystal glasses that were received as wedding and naming day gifts? And what about your many icons and religious trinkets? Though we have packed up your home so many times, there were still so many things left. Who would have thought that when you left Greece with a few suitcases, you would amass so much?

Family have taken things to remember you by. Dolores has taken an apron, some of the crystal platters, and some drinking glasses. It feels so joyous seeing her anticipatory excitement at starting her own household in years to come. Emmanuel took some icons and a model of the Acropolis. Cousin Jorge chose an icon and a small embroidery, has had them beautifully restored. I've given your jewellery box and a piece of jewellery to Kathy. Sophia has your ornate vigil candle that you lit each night. Cousin Konstantina took some of your nighties: she says they wrap her like a warm Chrisoula hug every time she wears them.

Your hand-tinted wedding photo now has pride of place in our living room. Your mixing bowls, oversized colander, and the trays you used to grind the dried oregano live in our pantry now. You always did everything big. When I use the colander, and

Epilogue

don your apron, I think of the many times we cooked together, of the beautiful legacy you have left me.

With all this 'doing' to help Dennis get into his new house and to pack up your home, my grief has threatened to overwhelm me at times. Though hard, it helps to visit people I can speak Greek with – your sisters, *Theia* Georgia, and my godmother – and share stories of you. We shed tears, are reminded of your goodness.

All these things keep me busy, along with working and looking after my own family, but there are times when I feel so fatigued that all I can do is scroll aimlessly through TikTok videos of someone mowing overgrown lawns, converting them into neat yards; or watching ovens being scrubbed free of their grime. There are days when I don't want to get out of bed. Days when I am so sapped of energy that I don't want to speak, want to retreat into my head and stay there. Random things catch me unawares, making me feel as if I'm being felled at the knees: seeing a recipe for potato salad that you used to make; overhearing a mother and daughter talking in Greek at the shops; seeing an image of you I haven't seen in a while.

I felt particularly vulnerable four months after you died. I told Dennis that I felt I had been doing a lot of carrying these past few years. And that I was scared I would now drop my bundle.

He'd looked confused. 'What bundle, Sis?'

I couldn't help but laugh. Dennis's life view seems so straightforward. Mum's pain was over. What was there to do now but move on? He has such a refreshing way of cutting through things.

Still, we all deal with things differently. My obsessive combing over of events in the small hours of the night scares me. I've done the sensible thing and met with a grief counsellor, who has encouraged me to write to you – not to say goodbye, but to say 'hello again'.

And so here I am, at your table, in the room that hosted so many parties. Almost all the cups have been cleared, the plates, all the tablecloths. These and the last of your furniture have been given away to support refugee families. Your clothes and your oversized sun hat have gone to itinerant farm workers. And even the recycled wrapping paper you collected so fastidiously has gone to wrap presents for charity Christmas sales. A woman from a local re-homing site helped me donate each of your precious things, talking us through it gently – did you send her by chance to make it easier for Dennis and me? I wouldn't put it past you. You would have loved that all your special things have gone to people who have very little.

I want to tell you how very much I miss you. How much I love you. I can't tell you that enough. Every remaining object, every surface, reminds me of you, but you are no longer here. I miss your calming, grounding presence. Your cheeky humour. I miss holding you, feeling your body soft and yielding in my arms.

You told me not to cry when you died, but we both knew that wasn't possible.

Epilogue

I dreamt of you the other night. We were talking, walking towards our old home in Collingwood. You were well. I knew our time together was limited, that you were just visiting, and that I must savour your being here. But you were not strong enough to make it all the way home, and I had to scoop you up in my arms to make the last leg. Soon we were in the living room, and I hugged you tightly, knowing you must go. And as you did, slipping down a crack into the earth below, I was left holding your clothes in my hands. In the murky shadows between sleep and wakefulness, I was filled with joy.

You wanted me to move on when you died, to look after my family. To look after myself, and my brother too. I am trying to do all those things. Working hard for them, and for you, to honour your beautiful memory. But still. You are not here.

I watch old home-videos of birthdays and naming days in a bid to remember you before you became so unwell. In them, you are always at the stove, or serving the next dish of food, imploring people to eat, to take more food home. You respond to everyone with ease, making them feel welcome. You barely have time to dance, but when you do, you do it wholeheartedly.

I remember how much preparation went into such big family events, and the stress of it in the lead up, but on the day, you are the consummate host, helping people be together, always making sure there was more than enough to eat. Your hands so busy with giving and making and nurturing.

Twelve Golden Gifts

I reflect on the gifts you have given us, your amazing legacy. I see this legacy in my cousins, who you treated like your own children. Your niece Georgia has inherited your strong faith, speaks to you each morning when she waters the orange tree you gave her, keeps a candle lit in your memory. Dim shares your father's name, and his, and your, infinite capacity for generosity and hard work. Jorge is keeping your grass edges straight until your home is sold, and rings Dennis daily. Kathy, who has opened her house to so many, makes sure that everyone who comes into her orbit is fed and welcome. Her daughter Sophia has your amazing capacity to see what needs to be done, and just does it. Dolores has inherited your earthy wisdom, and Emmanuel your empathy. And Dennis has your uncanny ability to listen wholeheartedly to everyone's story with an open heart, refusing to judge.

What have I inherited from you, *Mamma mou*? Do I have your ability to find the good in the bad, the light in the dark, and to wheedle out the laughter that might be hiding there? What I do know is that I always try to find the words that help build people up as you always did.

When I feel sad and lost, I stand in front of your photo in the hall, reminding myself of the gifts you gave us. *Mamma mou*, you are beside me when I cook, guiding my hands as I cut parsley and thyme and oregano from our own garden; when I stir it into the food that I cook for my family (more oil, Spiridoula, more oil!); when I wash our dishes and wipe my hands on the

Epilogue

apron that was yours. My hands haven't worked anywhere near as hard as yours, *Mamma mou*. But like yours, they are rarely still. I use them to write words in a bid to honour you. To share your irrepressible spirit so that you are not forgotten. I write them to keep you alive.

I've covered your table with a pretty tablecloth, as if you were here to see it. Soon, that too will go, but I will keep it as long as possible. I imagine you sitting here with us, surrounded by Emmanuel and Dolores, by Dennis and George. The kids have bought their partners. You are so excited, all anxious activity. What can I get you?!

I imagine time passing, and we are at a different table, in our own home. You are still sitting with us. Perhaps our grandkids have come to visit. You look so proud. You will try to push money into their little hands. You will encourage George to pick tomatoes from the garden to give to them, tell me that I should fry them up some chips.

More time passes, and in my mind's eye, you and I are sitting side by side at the table. We are both old. The children are spilling drinks, the adults telling stories. I smile at you, and you smile back. We are continuing the memories and bloodlines – and you, your irrepressible spirit, the gifts you have given us, are such a big part of it.

Mamma mou, I can see you as clearly as if you are here: your hands moving, your blue eyes twinkling.

Does everyone have enough to eat?

Twelve carer lessons

The following are twelve key lessons learnt as a carer and advocate for my mother. Some helped my brother and me support Mum at the time. Others were insights gleaned afterwards through talking to those with lived experience, as well as organisations working in the areas of dementia care, advocacy and carer support. Some of these insights would have been helpful to know at the time, particularly around managing Mum's pain, and on how to more effectively speak up when engaging with health and aged care systems. Though the learnings relate to our particular situation – especially as Mum's representatives when she could no longer advocate for herself – I hope that they might help others in similar situations.

It's important to remember that people with dementia can have decision-making capacity at almost all stages of the disease. As an advocate, it is key to keep your elder's best interests and wishes at the forefront of every decision made.

Twelve carer lessons

1. *Dementia is not one disease*

Dementia is a collection of diseases that affects the brain in different and complex ways. According to Dementia Australia, when someone has dementia, they have a 'disease of the brain which damages parts of it, stopping those parts working like they should. Dementia changes the way people think, feel and act'.

They state that dementia is not a normal part of getting older, and it isn't one specific disease. Instead, it's a broad term that covers the effects on people of a number of different medical conditions. Those conditions include Alzheimer's disease, vascular dementia, the Lewy body dementias and more.

Dementia Support Australia notes that, 'There are many reasons why the behaviour of a person with dementia can change. It may be due to physical changes in the brain. Or it could be caused by a person's environment, health or medication. Dementia can affect a person's ability to control how they respond to situations. Their behaviour may be the only thing they have left to communicate with.'

Educating yourself about the disease and its potential impacts on your loved one as it progresses and changes, can be empowering. Do this at your own pace, as too much information, and 'jumping ahead' to the later stages of the disease, can be overwhelming. Dementia Australia is a great starting point for information. They run free courses for family, carers and friends, and can refer you to organisations and websites for more information.

Twelve Golden Gifts

2. Celebrate and enjoy the small things

As Mum's disease progressed and it became so much harder to communicate with her, I found it helped to focus on taking pleasure in the small things – from sitting in the sunny courtyard of the care home, to massaging Mum's hands, to straightening a blanket across her knees. These are things she enjoyed when she was well and continued to enjoy in the last months and weeks of her life.

Even during the most challenging times when Mum seemed to be absent, it helped to remind myself that Mum *had a disease*, but she was *not her disease*. She was a person with many trials and joys amassed over a lifetime. She had very human frailties and flaws. She was still able to experience joy and pleasure and feel the warmth in our touch and voice. Though she could not express herself at all at the end, trying to step into her shoes and understanding what she needed at any given time helped both her, and us, feel like we could 'sit' with her and be helpful.

In the exquisitely poignant book *Dear Life*, about end-of-life care in a hospice environment, Dr Rachel Clark observes that even though her patients know they are dying, they often have the 'capacity to inhabit the present, in defiance of the future'.

3. Advocates can help keep elders' best interests in mind

Navigating the aged care and medical system as an elder with dementia without some sort of advocate, or advocates, I believe, would be incredibly hard. Often an advocate will be a family member or members who find they have to step up to troubleshoot problems, help fill in forms, and liaise with government departments, medical and residential care providers. Sometimes people such as health professionals, professional advocates and even third parties can help negotiate entry into systems such as aged care, or help to deal with conflict in hospital settings for example. There are patient advocates in most major hospitals. The Older Person's Advocacy Network (OPAN) has advocates to help address aged care service issues. These advocates can help talk through your concerns, point you to tools to help you self-advocate, and/or provide advocates to stand beside you in discussions with aged care services.

There are many things to think about as an advocate, but the main one in my mind was always how to walk the sometimes tricky line between supporting Mum so she could maintain independence, dignity and agency, while keeping her safe and comfortable. While these two things are not mutually exclusive, sometimes there was a conflict there.

Negotiating how to give her what she really wanted (to 'get her words back', to stay at home, to return home) versus what I perceived she most needed (to be safe, to be comfortable and pain free, to be close to people who loved her, to provide familiarity in language and food) was something that was often challenging. Still, at even the late stages of her disease, I tried to give her appropriate information in words I felt she would understand, get her opinion, and explain to her what was going to happen. I tried as much as possible to help her feel empowered within the limitations of her disease, and the settings in which she found herself.

4. Beware the administration

The administration involved in caring for and advocating for an elder, particularly an elder with dementia, needs to be experienced to be believed. Applying for, meeting about, and managing Home Care Packages, through the Commonwealth Government's My Aged Care website, organising enduring power of attorney and advanced care directives, and finding and negotiating the legal and financial issues around residential aged care, takes a lot of energy, time, and skill. Add to this trying to glean what your loved one wants and agrees to, and the many losses associated with dementia, and you've got a full plate.

You don't need to do it all alone. Delegate some things that aren't your area of expertise if you can. Get help and advice whenever possible. Draw on friends and family who have had good experiences and can recommend helpful supports and contacts, particularly for dealing with legal and financial matters. A surprising number of my peers were supporting, or had supported, elderly parents. They were often very glad to impart their own learnings and perceived fails. No one found it easy. I often find it very comforting to share and learn. Eventually I was able to pass on my own learnings.

Keeping a notebook and recording everything from Centrelink call reference and form numbers, to what elders say they want and need, will go a long way towards maintaining your sanity (thank you, Jean Kittson!). Don't be surprised if one notebook turns into two or more.

5. Ask questions

It seems almost too basic to state, but it's okay to ask questions of the many people that will likely be looking after your loved one. While we had many good experiences with those at the forefront of Mum's care, there were times when service providers spoke specialised language that we didn't understand.

While I didn't need to know every detail of Mum's care, those that impacted her quality of life – particularly around pain management and comfort – I felt it was important to ask about and understand. I find getting information powerful, and I can't help but ask questions. Some people prefer not to know. There is no right or wrong way to be.

If you do have questions, making them open-ended can help. For example:

It seems like this is happening ... what's your take on it?
Can you please explain it to me?
What are the options?
What are the implications of that?
I don't quite understand, can you please explain what that means?

If you don't understand something, or find yourself disagreeing with a course of action, then you have the right to clarify.

6. Be kind and respectful

It is not hard to experience strong emotions when the hold music on a government department helpline trills in your ear – one of the many frustrations when waiting in the queue to use the services of an under resourced and overwhelmed aged care and healthcare system. But it's a privilege to *have* such systems, complex and sluggish as they are at times. Personal care workers, call centre operators and aged care and hospital frontline staff should not have to bear the brunt of our frustration, grief or anger. The cleaners and personal carers in an aged care home are just as important as the chief executive officer – if not more so. As a visitor to residential care, you are entering not only the home of your loved one, but someone's workplace.

Treat the people who do the hard yards with our vulnerable elderly with kindness, empathy and respect. There is a big difference between being aggressive and assertively expressing what you need. Show that you are grateful to those looking after your loved one in whatever way you can.

7. Know what to expect

Aged care services should *give you what you need* in keeping with the Statement of Rights for older people within the *Aged Care Act 2024*.

Twelve carer lessons

This Statement provides a good reference point so that you can understand your rights as an elder, or a supporter of an elder.

A frank discussion about what is important to your elder, and what is possible, is a good one to have when requesting home care services and when in residential care. The Older Persons Advocacy Network has checklists to help identify what is important to elders, and on how to speak up when you are concerned about the delivery of your government aged care services.

In residential aged care, there are various key stages at which the discussions around your loved one's care can be had so that you can get some clarity on what you can expect from these services. These include:

- When choosing a residential home
- At the intake meeting prior to admission to the care home
- When transitioning from respite care to permanent car
- At any regular review meetings set up (generally every few months) to check in
- At any time that you feel a concern that adversely impacts your loved one's care needs to be raised.

You and/or your loved one have the right to request your loved one's care plan and to discuss how this is implemented.

A useful piece of advice I was given by a senior aged care worker was not to let the little concerns bank up – try and speak about them as they arise. I believe a good aged care provider will listen to your concerns, and work with you and your loved one to address them respectfully. They may not be able to meet all your expectations, but hopefully they will let you know why, and you can decide how you want to proceed accordingly.

If you are a decision maker for someone in residential aged care who can no longer make decisions for themselves, an excellent resource is the Dignified Respectful Decisions website, www.dard.org.au, created by Palliative Care Victoria. This provides clear and helpful information and support for people caring for a loved one, including how to prepare to be a decision maker, working together with the aged care team, working collaboratively as a decision maker and planning for end of life.

8. Speak up when things don't seem right

If it feels really wrong, then it probably is. This applies through the whole journey of caring for an elder – from responding if you think your loved one is acting uncharacteristically, to questioning care that doesn't seem helpful, dignified or safe.

Neglect and abuse are far too common in aged care, as identified by the Royal Commission into Aged Care Quality and Safety – these things need to be addressed at a systemic level. However, as a consumer of aged care services (or carers and advocates of those using those services), when you believe something is not right, *you're right to speak up without fear of reprisal.*

If you have a concern with your elder's care in a residential care facility, and if you feel comfortable, it's best to find out the right person to speak to and speak with them directly. Generally, this might be a nurse or the clinical manager. In a small facility, it might be the director or chief executive officer. If possible, take the time to speak to them when you are not angry or upset. If they agree to something relating to planning your loved one's care, follow up with an email thanking them and briefly outlining what was discussed. If you don't hear back within what you believe is a reasonable timeframe, then follow it up.

If you are not sure about how to speak up, with whom, or when, professional patient advocates in hospitals, and OPAN for example, can help.

9. Pain can, and should, be managed

So much of what we struggled with when it came to Mum's care was whether she was comfortable and pain free – from the time she fell at home and in hospital, to how much pain she experienced from pressure sores, to whether she was being turned regularly, as she could not do this herself. In the last few months of her life, the only way Mum could express her pain was by grimacing and moaning when turned. This is not uncommon in the later stages of dementia.

I have since been reminded that pain management is a fundamental human right. According to a report providing guidance on pain management in older people: 'Pain is not a normal part of the ageing process; however, chronic and persistent pain is common. Most residents living in residential aged care facilities have pain.'[1] A toolkit for managing pain in aged care states that 'People living in aged care who experience pain have the right to the acknowledgment of their pain and to be informed about how it can be assessed and managed by trained healthcare professionals.'[2]

As a layperson, I found it hard to know what questions to ask around pain management. It felt at the time that there were very few choices between mild pain management (think Panadol) to very heavy-duty opioids (think Endone/oxycodone), which have several side-effects.

If you or your loved one are concerned about pain, there are options for getting help. If caring at home, speak to your loved one's medical practitioner and other allied health workers (i.e. occupational therapist, physiotherapist) to discuss options available, and any potential side-effects.

If your loved one is in residential care, talk about any concerns around pain with the nurse or clinical manager who may be able to work with the GP, a geriatrician or pain specialist to come up with solutions. Some non-pharmaceutical measures such as compression stockings, heat packs and more frequent turning, may help.

---

[1] Abdulla A, Adams N, Bone M, et al. 'Guidance on the management of pain in older people'. *Age Ageing*. 2013; 42 Suppl 1:i1-57.

[2] Savvas S, Dang C, Peck A, Vaughan M & Scherer S.2021. *Pain Management Guide (PMG) Toolkit for Aged Care*, 2nd Edition. National Ageing Research Institute: Melbourne and Australian Pain Society, Sydney.

Palliative Care Australia suggests that having an open and honest conversation with your healthcare professional, whether that be your GP, your specialist, or your palliative care team, is a good start to assess and plan for pain management.

10. You can't help others if you can't care for yourself

By way of sustaining my own health and sanity as a carer, I tried to continue doing the simple things that gave me joy – going for a walk, cooking a meal, speaking to a friend. I encouraged my brother to do the same. Though I did these things less frequently and for a shorter duration, as caring, advocating and visiting Mum took up a lot of time, I kept doing them because they kept me going. I tried to keep close, the people I could really talk to. As Mum's disease progressed and became more challenging, this was a lifeline. I tried to ask for help where possible. I believe most people feel useful when they can help, even if only in a small way. When I felt that I was burdening my loved ones with my needs, particularly around grief after Mum had died, I sought professional help. Carers Australia notes that, 'It is well recognised that caring for someone with dementia can be one of the most demanding forms of care.' They write that caring:

- can be accompanied by feelings of loss and grief for the relationship and life you once shared with the person you are caring for

- can impact on relationships with family and friends who do not know how to react to your situation.

They go on to say that some behaviours exhibited by people with dementia can result in social stigma when you are out in the community and even with close friends or acquaintances.

Around three in four primary carers of people with dementia stated they had one or more physical or emotional effects due to the caring role. The most commonly reported impact was carers feeling weary or lacking energy, frequently feeling worried or depressed and having interrupted sleep.[3]

The option to access respite care to give us a break was explained to Dennis, Mum and I as part of Mum's initial aged care assessment. Like many, our response was that we wanted to do it all ourselves. What this meant is that Dennis became very fatigued and frustrated as the live-in carer. As Mum's disease progressed, it became increasingly challenging to meet her needs, even with both Dennis and me working together to manage her care.

Respite is a lifeline for many and may mean keeping your loved one at home for longer. Others treat it as a way of finding a suitable care home that meets their needs. Others access

---

[3] Australia Institute of Health and Welfare. 'Dementia in Australia web report', www.aihw.gov.au/reports/dementia/dementia-in-aus/contents/carers-and-care-needs-of-people-with-dementia/impact-of-the-caring-role-on-carers

it due to an emergency, or to make time to deal with their own health issues. There are different types of government-subsidised respite services available. This includes day and overnight respite and short stays in residential aged care homes. For more information about short-term respite care, see the My Aged Care website.

11. Messy feelings are part of caring

I don't think I speak just for myself when I say that messy feelings are part and parcel of caring for someone with dementia – particularly guilt, anger and shame.

Dr Karen Hitchcock, in her book *Dear Life* about the treatment of our elderly in Australian hospitals, says of her patients, 'No one wants to go into a nursing home. My patients fear it; families often feel terrible guilt when the time comes; it is thought of as an abandonment.'

There are a lot of supports and information on how to acknowledge and work through feelings of guilt, shame and grief. The basic tips below are just a starting point.

If you're a carer, be kind to yourself. Do the best you can. Step away when it gets too much, even briefly. If you find you are getting physically or mentally unwell, or are unable to manage anger, get the help you need to see you through. You can't look after someone if you yourself are unwell.

There are lots of places to get help and support, including your GP, Dementia Australia and the Carer Gateway.

12. Allow yourself to grieve

'Grief is fundamental to our humanity. Grieving for the loss of someone, or anticipating the loss of someone, is something that gives our life value. It means that we've loved people, and they've loved us,' says comedian Jean Kittson.

'Grief is the form love takes when someone dies,' writes Dr Rachel Clarke in *Dear Life*.

The winner of the SBS program *Alone Australia* 2023, the charismatic Gina Chick, says of her own grief at the loss of her young daughter that it came in waves, bubbled up and moved through her like a strong wind. She says she learnt to be present for her grief, that she accepted that it needed to be felt rather than pushed away. In short, she said 'yes' to her grief and to the journey that it took her on.

Reading and hearing these words helped me affirm my intuition that I needed to work *with* my grief rather than *against* it. I've tried not to fight the messiness and seeming madness of my grief. At times it's taken hold of my body and hurt in a very visceral way. I've learnt to move with it because I know intuitively that if I try and push against it, or bullishly fight it, it will just come back to bite me later on.

Grieving is part of the human condition. Let yourself wail or swear if you have to. Talk and write to your loved one while they are still alive, and afterwards too. Do what helps with the sadness and tragedy of seeing someone you love decline. There is no right or wrong way to do this thing. Often when caring for someone with dementia, the grief starts at diagnosis – it is usually a very slow burn. There is no timeline for grief: you don't just get 'over it' or 'move on' after the first few weeks, months, or even years after someone dies – it seems to just become a part of you and the fabric of your being. So often grief feels like such a lonely process, and riding the waves can be hard work, particularly if it's difficult to find outlets to express it. Though sometimes challenging, talk with those who will listen and sit with your grief. If you don't have those people in your own networks, there are many online options for support – it's astounding how many people are out there experiencing grief. Finally, seek professional help if your grief is impacting your life in unhelpful ways. Your GP and organisations such as Grief Australia and Griefline are a good starting point.

More information

CARER GATEWAY

Carer Gateway is a Commonwealth Government initiative with a national network of providers who help carers access in-person, phone and online support services.

How they can help

- free online and phone counselling for carers
- carer wellbeing fact sheets
- information on services available to support carers, including peer support groups, support packages, skills courses, coaching, and information/access to emergency respite.

Contact

☎ 1800 422 737 (Freecall, 8am–5pm weekdays, 24/7 for emergency respite)

💻 carergateway.gov.au

DEMENTIA AUSTRALIA

There are many sources of information about dementia, but a good starting point is Dementia Australia. They are the national peak body supporting people living with dementia, their families and carers. In 2024, it is estimated that more than 421,000 Australians live with dementia. Dementia is the second leading cause of death of all Australians. More than 1.6 million people in Australia are involved in the care of someone living with dementia. Dementia Australia offers information, advice and support, no matter what your experience of dementia.

How they can help

- free National Dementia Helpline 24 hours a day, seven days a week, 365 days a year
- confidential information, advice and support on dementia and memory loss concerns for yourself and others
- free online and in-person information sessions for carers and family
- written resources on many aspects of dementia care
- referral to organisations and professionals who can help with your particular situation.

Contact

☎ National Dementia Helpline: 1800 100 500 (Freecall, 24/7)
💻 www.dementia.org.au

More information

DEMENTIA SUPPORT AUSTRALIA

Dementia Support Australia is a national, free 24/7 telephone service that helps people with dementia where changed behaviours are impacting their lives or the lives of their carer.

How they can help

- dedicated helpline 24 hours a day, seven days a week
- specialised dementia consultants work out which service will be most suitable based on individual circumstances and impact of behaviour change
- personalised strategies, advice and practical ways to support the person in your care.

Contact

☎ 24-Hour help 1800 699 799

💻 www.dementia.com.au

GRIEF AUSTRALIA

Grief Australia is an independent, not for profit organisation, providing counselling, training, and research.

How they can help

- free counselling (online and in-person)
- support groups for anyone experiencing a loss due to death (in-person and online)
- support and resources for professionals.

Contact

☎ 1800 642 066 (Freecall, 9am–5pm weekdays)

💻 www.grief.org.au

GRIEFLINE

Griefline is dedicated to helping individuals navigate the complexities of grief and loss. They provide free, accessible support and resources to people across Australia.

How they can help

- free telephone support and resources
- bereavement support groups
- 24/7 online forums

Contact

☎ 1300 845 745 (Freecall, 8am–8pm, 7 days a week)

💻 griefline.org.au

MY AGED CARE

My Aged Care is a starting point for accessing Australian Government-funded aged care services. It provides information and support to understand, access and navigate the aged care system.

How they can help

Give information on what aged care services are available, information on costs, and how you can apply for these, including:

- services available in the home, such as cleaning, shopping, bathing etc.
- short-term and respite care
- information on aged care homes and options.

Contact

You can access My Aged Care online, on the phone or in person.

☎ 1800 200 422 (Freecall, 8am–8pm weekdays; 10am–2pm Saturdays)

💻 www.myagedcare.gov.au

More information

OLDER PERSONS ADVOCACY NETWORK

The Older Persons Advocacy Network (OPAN) is a national network of nine non-profit organisations that provides free, confidential and independent information and support to older people seeking or receiving government-funded aged care as well as their families and other representatives.

How they can help

- information on aged care rights
- easy-to-use self-advocacy toolkits
- decision-making resources and tools
- advocates available for information or support
- advice on what to do when things go wrong in aged care.

Contact

☎ 1800 700 600 (Freecall, 8am–8pm weekdays; 10am–4pm Saturdays)

💻 opan.org.au

Permissions

The following published stories have been adapted here.

'The gift from Mum's Cypriot watchmaker', SBS Voices, 27 June 2022

'Going through my parent's possessions reminded me of the sacrifices they made', SBS Voices, 9 September 2020

'Cooking for my mother now that she can no longer do it herself', SBS Voices, 21 October 2020

Acknowledgements

To my publisher Mary Rennie and her team at ABC Books/HarperCollins, thank you for seeing the potential of *Twelve Golden Gifts*, and for making the leap of faith that my words might resonate with a bigger audience. To brilliant editors Kathy Hassett and Lachlan McLaine, for treating our story with such respect. To my literary agent Jacinta di Mase, thank you for your support and encouragement over more than 15 years – I'm ever grateful for your continued championing of so many authors' work.

To the many people who provided formal care for Mum – from physios to nurses, from personal carers to doctors – with particular thanks to Mum's GP, Dr John Kondopoulos. Special thanks too to organisations Dementia Australia, Elder Rights Australia, Grief Australia and Palliative Care Victoria for their review and input into the resources and practical learnings of this book.

To the family friends who I grew up with and who are still such a big part of my supportive 'village': Tina Tasiopoulos, Konstantina Vlahos, Gina Christo, Fiona Samios, Litsa Patterson and Mary Hartley in particular.

There are too many friends to mention individually here, but a special thanks goes to friends Sarah-Jane Mead, Robyn Cole Selleck and Jane Anderson, who listened so generously, and who helped in very practical ways to plan Mum's funeral. To Maria and Kalliopi Tzikas who provided guidance on religious rituals towards the end of Mum's life – thank you. To Mum's beautiful neighbours Brigitte and Adam Kurowski, who delivered so many meals. To my friend Julie Hassard for her many gentle conversations about end-of-life care, and on the importance of treasuring each day. To my sister-in-law Josephine who has done so much heavy lifting when it comes to her folks – thanks for being such an amazing model.

To my in-laws Alfred and Doris, thank you for your continued love and support. Papa, may your beautiful spirit soar.

To my writer's group – Myfanwy Jones, Sam Lawry, Maryrose Cuskelly and Wendy Meddings – thanking you for years of support, encouragement and wise counsel, and for walking alongside me with this work.

To my colleagues Jacqui Ross, Timothy Richards, Amanda Apthorpe and Nicolas Brasch thank you for your generosity in reading the first draft of this book and for your sustained

Acknowledgements

encouragement. What a blessing to work with such a great team to teach and talk about stories and books.

To my cousins Katerina Petras, Dimmy Tsimiklis, Georgia Iliadis and Jorge Onasis, and to Aunty Sofia and my nieces and nephews who helped with advice, meals, gardening, and even fixing taps so they were easy for Mum to manage! Ever grateful for your ongoing love and support.

To our children Dolores and Emmanuel – so proud of the wonderful young adults you have become, and sorry about having way too many dinner conversations about elderly parents. Yiayia loved you to the moon and back and has left you the most amazing legacy.

To my husband George Mifsud, who provides the morning coffee, the hugs and the debriefs. It's been a hard journey caring for three elderly parents over several years, but we still managed to find the laughter and silliness (most days).

To my brother Dennis Tsintziras, who has given me the gift of trust to tell our story. I am so grateful to you for taking on Mum's day-to-day care for so long. I look forward to more sunny tomorrows.

Finally, to my mother Chrisoula – my muse, my angel – this book is my love letter to you, my way of honouring your irrepressible golden spirit. I hope my meagre words do you justice. You will never be forgotten. *Aionia I mnimi sou.* May your memory be eternal.